YOGA RX

LARRY PAYNE, PH.D., AND

RICHARD USATINE, M.D.

Edited By Merry Aronson

and Rachelle Gardner

Broadway Books NEW YORK

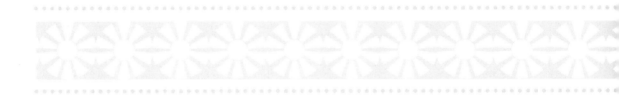

YOGA RX

A Step-by-Step Program

to Promote Health, Wellness,

and Healing for Common Ailments

To Merry, with love.

L.P.

To Moira, a loving sister

and a wonderful mother.

R.U.

YOGA RX. Copyright © 2002 by Larry Payne, Ph.D., and Richard Usatine, M.D. All rights reserved. No part of this book may be reproduced or transmitted in any form or by any means, electronic or mechanical, including photocopying, recording, or by any information storage and retrieval system, without written permission from the publisher. For information, address Broadway Books, a division of Random House, Inc., 1540 Broadway, New York, NY 10036.

PRINTED IN THE UNITED STATES OF AMERICA

Broadway Books titles may be purchased for business or promotional use or for special sales. For information, please write to: Special Markets Department, Random House, Inc., 1540 Broadway, New York, NY 10036.

BROADWAY BOOKS and its logo, a letter B bisected on the diagonal, are trademarks of Broadway Books, a division of Random House, Inc.

Visit our Web site at www.broadwaybooks.com

Library of Congress Cataloging-in-Publication Data

Payne, Larry.
Yoga Rx : a step-by-step program to promote health, healing and wellness / Larry Payne and Richard Usatine.
p. cm.
Includes index.
1. Yoga, Haòha. 2. Healing. 3. Health. I. Usatine, Richard. II. Title.

RA781.7 .P395 2002
613.7'046--dc21
2002074781

ISBN 0-7679-0749-3

FIRST EDITION

Designed by Dana Leigh Treglia
Illustrated by Kathryn Hewitt
Photographs by Blaine Michioka

3   5   7   9   10   8   6   4

Contents

Acknowledgments

We would like to express our appreciation for the many people who made this book possible.

Special thanks to Rebecca Cole, our editor at Broadway Books, for her wisdom, patience, and guidance, and to Dana Treglia for the beautiful design of this book. We are grateful for the enormous talent of Rachelle Gardner, who helped us find our voice and continuously gave invaluable assistance. Our technical editors Richard Rosen and Art Brownstein, M.D., helped us keep our facts straight, and our extraordinary photographer, Blaine Michioka, captured the beauty of Yoga in pictures. We thank our undaunted literary agent, Carol Susan Roth, and the consultants and friends who gave selflessly of their time and knowledge: Sri Mishra, M.D.; Richard Miller, Ph.D.; Robert Forster, P.T.; Roger Cole, Ph.D.; David Allen, M.D.; James Galizia, M.D.; Mike Sinel, M.D.; Lesly Kaminoff; Kausthub Desikachar; Linda Lack, M.A.; Judy Gantz, M.A.; Leroy Perry, D.C.; Steve Paredes, D.C.; Professor Sasi Velupillai; John Schumacher; Joseph Le Page; Roberta Haas; Shinzen Young;

Ron Lawrence, M.D.; Leslie Bogart, R.N.; David and Karen McHugh; Marc Suchard; Ram Rao, M.D.; Matra Majmundar, O.T.R.; Brother Keshavananda; Erick Maisel; Clark Siegel; Chris Brisco; and Ingrid Kelsey. For editorial assistance and research we thank Lauren Marino; Stephan Bodian, Ph.D.; Trisha Lamb Feuerstein; David Hurwitz; Marguerite Baca; Suzi Landolphi; and Kathryn Hewitt for illustrations. Thanks also to models Karen Howard (cover), Randi Jo Greenberg, and Laura Dunning, and stylists Jeanne Townsend and JoJo Meyers Proud. We especially appreciate the dedicated staff of Broadway Books who made this book a reality.

FROM LARRY PAYNE:

My deepest gratitude to T. K. V. Desikachar for his inspiration and example. To my immediate family: Dolly, Harold, Chris, Lisa, James, Natalie, and Maria. To my legal counsel and friend Steve Ostrow, and my personal assistant Chris Fletcher. To my beloved teachers who guide my spiritual path: Parmahansa Yogananda; Evarts Loomis, M.D.; Indra Devi; Georg Feuerstein, Ph.D.; Richard Miller, Ph.D.; Lilias Folan; and Rama Vernon. To all my Yoga students and Yoga therapy clients whose courage inspires me. And finally, I thank God for my friendship with Richard Usatine. It has been an honor to work on this project together.

FROM DR. RICHARD USATINE:

Special thanks to Larry for his friendship and for giving me the tools and the encouragement to heal my back pain. I'm also deeply grateful that he devoted himself to creating and teaching the first class on Yoga and Medicine for UCLA medical students. Finally, I would like to thank Larry for conceiving of this book and asking me to be his partner. I am pleased that we were able to present the ancient art of Yoga in a context that stays true to current scientific principles.

I would like to thank my lovely wife, Janna, and my wonderful children, Rebecca and Jeremy, for their support and love. My family brings joy to my life every day and gives meaning to my work.

A Note from Larry

and Richard

The doctor of the future will give no medicine,
but will interest his patient in the care of the human frame,
in dict and in the cause and prevention of disease.
—*Thomas A. Edison*

Yoga has dramatically changed both our lives. We wrote this book because we wanted to help you restore your health, relieve your pain, and feel better through Yoga therapy.

As a Yoga therapist and a medical doctor, we have different backgrounds and lead very diverse lives. Yet both of us have experienced such powerful effects from Yoga that we have committed ourselves to sharing this extraordinary healing tool with others. We believe Yoga is one of the most effective ways to treat your body and mind simultaneously, reducing stress and increasing flexibility, muscle strength, concentration, and a general sense of well-being. We want to spread the news that Yoga is not only effective for overall health, it can also be used in a targeted manner, with specially designed postures and routines, to manage and even cure specific physical disorders.

As part of his medical practice, Dr. Richard Usatine teaches the basics of Yoga to patients suffering from ailments as varied as back pain, anxiety, and asthma. He refers many patients to Yoga therapy for healing of their painful and injured bodies. Dr. Larry Payne is a Yoga teacher and therapist working each week with hundreds of people, in classes and in one-on-one therapy sessions, to improve their health.

A few words about our backgrounds before we met will help you understand how we both became so passionate about Yoga.

RICHARD'S STORY

I took my first Yoga class when I was in college and was wary because I thought I'd be spending a lot of time sitting in the lotus position, a popular image back in the 1970s. I was relieved to find that the postures of Yoga are many and varied—and they feel great. I saw how Yoga could help me increase my flexibility and learn to relax both my mind and my body. Since then, I have used Yoga intermittently with other physical activities, including swimming, cycling, squash, and tennis.

After medical school, I completed my family medicine residency at the University of California at Los Angeles (UCLA) and then practiced full-time at the Venice Family Clinic. From the beginning, I took a holistic approach to treating patients. I listened to their stories, made house calls, and developed strong relationships with the patients and their communities. Meanwhile, the medical students and residents I was training at the clinic learned the value of caring for the whole person, taking into account their physical, mental, and emotional needs.

In 1989, I returned to UCLA to co-direct the family medicine training program for interns and residents. Influenced by holistic ideas in the works of Bernie Siegel, Joan Borysenko, and John Sarno, I began to teach mind–body medicine to residents. The idea was to get young doctors to promote an overall healthy lifestyle to their patients. Meanwhile, furthering my study of Yoga gave me an opportunity to learn more about the mind–body connection and the value of Yoga in my own life. One instance of this was when I was able to use Yoga to heal a skiing injury to my knee. I began referring my own patients to Yoga for various conditions, both physical and stress related, and I constantly received positive feedback on Yoga's effects.

In 1990, I began teaching doctors how to help their patients quit smoking through abdominal breathing, the same Yoga breathing I had learned many years before. Patients were able to cope with the stress and anxiety of quitting their addiction, and we had quite a success rate! This was just one of the countless medically sound uses I have found for Yoga in my years as a family physician and a teacher.

LARRY'S STORY

In 1978, I was an advertising sales executive living in Los Angeles and working for a major New York–based women's magazine. The money was great, and the perks were even better. I drove a fancy company car, had a generous expense account, and enjoyed my work. But, as the advertising business became more competitive, the pressure intensified and I became totally overwhelmed. Eventually, I developed high blood pressure and a serious back problem. For the next two years, my job-related stress continued while doctors tried to fix my back. Orthopedic specialists, physical therapists, and prescription drugs all failed to bring relief. The only options left were surgery, more drugs, or learn to live with it.

Then a dear friend virtually dragged me (not quite kicking and screaming; I was willing to try anything) to a Yoga class. I remember being embarrassed, thinking I couldn't possibly do those strange postures the right way. My muscles were tight, and I was wired from the stress of my job. Fortunately, the teacher was compassionate and wise. She instructed me in the postures and the Yoga breathing, advising me not to be competitive or to push myself too hard. At the end of the class, she led us in a guided relaxation for about ten minutes. I couldn't believe it. The pain in my back disappeared for the first time in two years. The relief lasted several hours, and I had this unfamiliar feeling of being relaxed and happy. It was a life-changing experience, and I was eager to share it with everyone around me.

I began to pursue the Yoga path seriously, first attending a Yoga and health retreat founded by Dr. Evarts Loomis, father of holistic medicine in America. Then I took a one-year sabbatical to study Yoga. My sojourn led me to eleven countries and eventually to India, the birthplace of Yoga. There I trained as a Yoga teacher and had the fortune to study with many of India's foremost Yoga masters, including my teacher of twenty years, T. K. V. Desikachar.

Well, that was it for advertising. When I returned to Los Angeles in 1981, I retired from the advertising world, became a full-time Yoga teacher, and founded the Samata Yoga Center. For the past two decades, I have worked to bring Yoga and Yoga therapy into the mainstream as a legitimate and respected health-care alternative.

OUR COLLABORATION

The two of us first met in 1997. A year earlier, Richard had been a passenger in an auto accident, and shortly afterward, the nagging low back pain began. Months later when the pain hadn't disappeared, he finally went for medical attention. The orthopedic doctors performed x-rays, computed tomography (CT) scans, magnetic resonance imaging (MRI), and even a bone scan, but they found nothing structural to explain the pain. Eventually, he was referred to Larry for Yoga therapy. At that first appointment, Larry took a history and assessed Richard's posture, flexibility, and gait. Larry developed a Yoga program specifically for Richard, and within a few short weeks Richard was essentially pain free and feeling completely well for the first time in more than a year. To this day, Richard uses the program Larry developed to keep his back flexible and healthy. (In Chapter 8, you will find a similar program, called Yoga for the Back.)

As we continued to work together, we began to discuss how valuable it would be for medical students to be exposed to Yoga, both for their own well-being and to provide them with a technique for their patients. Together, we created an elective class in Yoga and Yoga therapy at the UCLA School of Medicine. In an innovative alliance of Western medicine and ancient Eastern philosophies, the course became an immediate success, and in 1998 it became a regular part of the school's elective curriculum—a first for a U.S. medical school. Larry teaches the theories of Yoga for one hour and leads the students in practicing Yoga for a second hour. Yoga now helps these students manage their stress and exposes them to Yoga as a beneficial therapy for their own future patients. It was exciting to observe a student from our first Yoga class teaching a patient how to use Yoga breathing and postures to overcome his back pain.

YOGA: NO PAIN, ALL GAIN

As most people know by now, there are vast quantities of scientific evidence showing that exercise enhances your health and prevents illness. The benefits of physical activity are cumulative, so that small amounts of time spent exercising on a regular and long-term basis will add up to big rewards. According to the Centers for Disease Control and Prevention (CDC), exercise:

- Increases muscle and bone strength.
- Increases lean muscle and decreases body fat.
- Helps control your weight.
- Enhances your psychological well-being and plays a part in reducing the development of depression.
- Reduces symptoms of anxiety and improves your general mood.

Yoga provides all of the benefits of exercise and more. The Yoga postures involve stretching to maintain and enhance flexibility. Many poses are a form of isometric strengthening exercise, which involve the contraction of muscles without moving the joint. In other words, you're working very hard to remain motionless. This technique, which strengthens muscles without putting too much stress on the joint, is often used in physical therapy for the rehabilitation of injured joints. Other Yoga poses involve movement, which is always done slowly and with focus. Because Yoga is safe and gentle, it can be enjoyed late into life, when normal aging causes many of us to lose flexibility and strength, making us more susceptible to injury.

But Yoga is more than just the physical movements and postures. The central element is Yoga breathing, which we encourage you to practice before you begin trying the routines. Yoga breathing simply means using various techniques to breathe in a slow and focused manner, which calms your mind and relaxes your body. More than twenty-five years ago Herbert Benson, a Harvard physician, researched the physiology of what he called our "relaxation response." He found that high blood pressure could be reduced with abdominal breathing and simple meditation. The relaxation breathing stimulates the parasympathetic nervous system, which is responsible for telling our bodies to relax. The vagus nerve is a part of this system; and when it is stimulated, it reduces the heart rate and the intensity of the heart pump, thereby lowering blood pressure. Although he did not specifically use Yoga techniques, the slow and measured breathing that went with the meditation he taught was identical to Yoga breathing. That does not mean that all people with high blood pressure can be treated exclusively with this type of breathing and the relaxation response. But Dr. Benson found that this was sufficient therapy for some patients and was beneficial for those patients who still needed medication. The benefits of Yoga breathing are numerous, and we'll go into them in detail in Chapter 5 and provide you with instructions and exercises.

There is overwhelming scientific evidence that the severity of many medical problems increases with stress. For example, virtually all types of pain worsen when a person is under great stress. We feel pain when our body sends pain messages to the brain through the spinal cord. When the brain is performing optimally, it sends blocking signals down the spinal cord, which decrease the transmission of pain to the central nervous system. When the brain is under stress, it appears that these blocking signals don't work as well so we experience pain more intensely. Stress can also exacerbate high blood pressure and lead to a heart attack. Yoga has the wonderful benefit of reducing stress through the relaxation response, plus it offers all the advantages of exercise.

Like all forms of exercise, Yoga should be performed only to your capacity. There are always exceptions; but if you are older, you should not expect to be as flexible and strong as younger people. It is essential that when you initially practice Yoga, you avoid pushing yourself beyond your limit. You cannot "muscle" your way into Yoga. Injuries occur when you try to force your body to do something your body is not prepared to do. Advocates of no pain—no gain will find no supporters here. The sensible, noncompetitive, and individualistic approach to Yoga should bring you nothing but increased flexibility, strength, and improved health— no matter where you start.

How to Use This Book

Yoga Rx is not meant to replace modern medical treatment, nor does this book attempt to supersede your doctor's diagnosis. We intend you to use it as a complement to other medical treatments, with the approval of your physician.

We urge you to read Parts I and II to get a basic understanding of Yoga therapy, before jumping to the chapter that contains your ailment. It's important that once you begin using Yoga to help relieve your condition, you practice with an understanding of the breathing, relaxation, and meditation techniques involved, as well as the basic principles of how Yoga heals. All of this is explained in Chapters 1 to 5. In Chapter 6, you will find two basic Yoga therapy routines that you can easily learn and practice when you are ready for general conditioning.

In Part III, you'll find common medical problems grouped according to the bodily system they belong to. For example, if you're interested in Yoga for back or knee pain, you should go to Chapter 7. Be sure to start at the beginning of the chapter, to learn how ancient Yoga philosophy and modern medicine come together to provide a thorough understanding of your condition. Each chapter explains the anatomical system, discusses different ailments of that system, describes how and why Yoga can enhance the health of the individual dealing with those problems, and illustrates ailment-specific Yoga therapy routines.

Throughout the book, we use real-life stories of people whose health has improved through Yoga. These anecdotes are not meant to be proof that Yoga will work for all people with similar ailments or disorders. However, they do illustrate the possibilities and we hope they encourage you to adopt healthier living practices, as some of our clients have done with Yoga and other lifestyle modifications.

If followed correctly, the recommendations in this book are safe for everyone. Because each individual is unique, people respond and improve at different rates. However, you can expect to notice considerable results within a couple weeks of beginning Yoga therapy and significant changes within three months.

Throughout the book, Larry addresses you in the first person as he relates anecdotes from his experience and his Yoga therapy practice. However, all of the medical and scientific information has been provided by Richard. You may not hear Richard's voice, but his medical expertise is on every page.

We have seen thousands of women and men make tremendous strides in their health, careers, and relationships through a regular practice of Yoga. We have also seen Yoga therapy bring about amazing improvements for longtime sufferers of back pain, hypertension, chronic fatigue syndrome, depression, asthma, allergies, arthritis, and numerous other maladies.

We have collaborated on this book in hopes that you will find not only relief from your pain and generally improved health but an appreciation of your body's ability to naturally heal itself when given the right conditions. It is our sincere wish that you will be able to use our concrete suggestions to improve your health and to experience a life of vitality, energy, and fulfillment through the art and science of Yoga therapy.

Larry Payne, Ph.D., and Richard Usatine, M.D.

YOGA RX

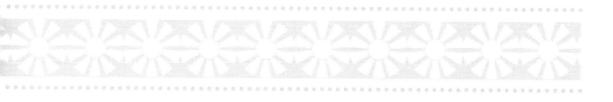

PART I

Introduction to Yoga Therapy

Part I of *Yoga Rx* introduces you to Yoga and, specifically, Yoga therapy. It's crucial for you to read these chapters to prepare yourself for learning the exercises in Parts II and III. Even if you're familiar with Yoga, you may be surprised at some of the new information you'll find here.

1

How Yoga Heals

Yoga is not magic, but it can bring about miraculous types of transformation. Jessica, nineteen, had been diagnosed with an assortment of ailments from her early teens. They included mononucleosis, chronic fatigue syndrome, hypothyroidism, severe allergies, and adrenal deficiency. Despite treatment and medication from three prominent doctors, she was unable to participate in normal physical activities without ending up in bed with flu-like symptoms. Her dismal health also affected her attitude about life, and she often found herself depressed and unhappy.

Unable to physically endure a group Yoga class, Jessica began private Yoga therapy lessons. She started with simple reclining breath and movement routines (similar to the Lower Back Routine, described on page 114). After a month, Jessica was able to intensify her practice and use Core Routine I (page 62). She started to have more energy for everyday activities that we take for granted when we are healthy. After three months, she had stopped taking most of her medications, could participate in normal activities, and had graduated to Core Routine II (page 78). Perhaps most important, her spirits had lifted, and she felt happy and hopeful for the first time in years.

"After a year of Yoga therapy, I had developed a two-hour daily routine," she recalls. "It included one hour of Yoga, forty-five minutes of treadmill, and fifteen minutes of Yoga breathing exercises—a regimen that would have previously been impossible for me to maintain." Using the principles of Yoga therapy, Jessica had succeeded in reclaiming her good health and a vital, energetic life.

So what is Yoga, anyway? Yoga is not just stretching, just breathing, or just meditation. It is not just crossing your legs, closing your eyes, putting your thumbs and forefingers together and chanting "Om . . ." And it is certainly not a cult or a religion.

I like to describe Yoga as a natural, do-it-yourself prescription for good health and stress management that is needed now more than ever in our demanding, stress-filled lives. Since modern medicine points to stress as a major cause of illness today, Yoga may ultimately prove to be one of the most practical preventative medicine techniques available. It has an illustrious five-thousand-year history, and since the 1970s its popularity in the West has skyrocketed.

Yoga is rightly considered an art. Similar to a dance that is carefully choreographed, Yoga consists of specific postures, techniques, and attitudes. Yet it's the individual performer who breathes life into the form, making the expression his or her own and transforming the routine into an art.

At the same time, Yoga is also a science. It is based on ancient observations, principles, and theories of the mind–body connection, many of which are now being discovered in medical research. Qualified teachers have passed down this precise knowledge to their students from one generation to the next. Often these teachers have been referred to as Gurus, meaning "the ones who remove darkness."

Yoga focuses on healing the whole person and views the mind and body as an integrated unity, which is why it is called a mind–body science. It teaches that, given the right tools and the right environment, the mind–body can find harmony and heal itself. Like an orchestra and its conductor, the systems of the body need to be in sync with the mind to perform effectively. If the mind provides confusing signals or moves too fast, the body may become imbalanced, out of sync, overworked, or exhausted. And if the systems of the body are weak or out of tune, they may not be able to respond to the mind. Yoga calms and relaxes the mind, strengthens and tunes the body, and brings them into harmony with one another.

Translated from Sanskrit, the classical language of India, the word *Yoga* means "yoke" or "unity." It also means "discipline" or "effort." In other words, Yoga requires you to make an *effort* to *unify* your body and mind. You do this by concentrating your awareness on your physical body. Many people think of Yoga as simply stretching or gymnastics. But unlike other exercise programs, you can't do Yoga postures properly while watching your favorite sitcom on TV. At the health club, you see people wearing headphones or reading the newspaper while they exercise. This is a perfect example of the mind attending to something else while the body is exercising. Because Yoga requires the full exertion of both the mind and the body, by definition it can't be practiced while your attention is elsewhere.

YOGA POSTURES

When most people hear the word *Yoga,* they picture a room full of people practicing the familiar postures known as asanas (AH-sah-nas). The approach to Yoga that focuses on these postures is called Hatha (HAHT-hah) Yoga and is generally taught in a group setting, rather than one to one. But there are other categories of Yoga that don't involve postures at all.

For example, Bhakti Yoga emphasizes loving devotion to a personal god, whereas Karma Yoga consists of selfless service. Jnana Yoga cultivates higher wisdom as a path to the divine, while Raja Yoga encourages the classical practice of meditation and contemplation. Mantra Yoga uses sacred sounds, or mantras, as a means of spiritual refinement, and Guru Yoga advocates dedication to a Yoga master. Each is a kind of Yoga because it involves self-discipline and seeks to "unite" the practitioner with the sacred dimension of being. In fact, even the Hatha Yoga we now associate with Yoga studios and rigorous routines was originally developed as a method for channeling spiritual energies and achieving higher states of consciousness.

Within Hatha Yoga itself there are many styles and lineages. Some of the more traditional approaches that have become well established in the United States include Iyengar, Ashthanga, Integral, Sivananda, Bikram, Ananda, Kundalini, and Kripalu. A number of Western teachers have developed their own unique styles as well, including Somatic, Hidden Language, White Lotus, Tri, Ishta, Anusara, and Jivamukti. In my practice, I use a style I call User Friendly Yoga™, which is my own slight modification of a traditional approach called Viniyoga. This is what you will find in the Yoga routines in this book.

According to one source, more people are enrolled in group Yoga classes in California than in the entire country of India. In 2001, *Yoga Journal* estimated that there were more than eleven million people practicing Yoga in the United States and approximately twenty million worldwide. Of all the locations in the world, I'm sure that none has more Hatha Yoga classes than Los Angeles. However, not all Yoga studios are created equal.

While researching this book I discovered a startling array of classes offered under the name *Yoga* within a five-mile radius of my Los Angeles studio. I attended one huge class with more than fifty students, in a sweltering room in which the temperature was over one hundred degrees and the teacher sported a bikini and used a headphone mike. Just up the street, the teachers were wearing long robes and burning incense, and chanting seemed to be the order of the day.

A few miles north, I found a studio with a hard wooden floor, straps hanging from the walls (don't ask!), and props such as blocks, benches, and blankets every-where. The teacher had the demeanor of a drill sergeant and yelled at his students as he inspected their postures. Finally, I ended up in a trendy center where the instructor was as funny as a stand-up comedian, rap music played throughout the class, and the students were bouncing and grooving as they practiced their poses. Only in America.

If you decide to venture into a Yoga class, it's important to do a little research first. Make sure the one you select fits your individual needs based on your fitness, age, state of mind, and overall energy level.

THE YOGA LIFESTYLE

Classical Yoga includes eight principles, which were described in detail in the second century B.C. in the *Yoga Sutras* of Pantanjali. The eight principles offer guidelines for a moral and meaningful existence, emphasizing moderation and self-discipline, which can be found in all of the world's great religions:

- ✳ Treat others as you would like to be treated; avoid violence in word and action.
- ✳ Work on your self-discipline to exchange bad habits for good ones.
- ✳ Maintain a practice of Yoga.
- ✳ Practice Yoga breathing techniques.
- ✳ Avoid overstimulation of the senses.
- ✳ Develop focus and concentration.
- ✳ Include meditation in your lifestyle.
- ✳ Work toward a goal of joy and ecstasy.

The practice of Yoga has a way of seeping into other parts of your life. For most people, it helps cultivate greater awareness; slows down the pace and increases enjoyment of simple, everyday activities; and generally improves their outlook.

Yoga will help you become more aware of your body's posture, alignment, and movement patterns, which in turn can have a powerful impact on how you feel. As you begin a Yoga practice, you may also notice that your internal rhythms slow down and your ability to concentrate improves. Systematic focus on breath and movement helps you tune into a deeper awareness of yourself and your surroundings.

As you maintain the more physical aspects of yoga, such as postures and breathing, you may also find yourself naturally drawn to change your lifestyle in accordance with these principles. Many of my students have reported that they gave up smoking or stopped eating junk food or meat after they had been practicing Yoga for a few months. In my experience, the more attuned you become to your body, the harder it becomes to treat yourself with disrespect.

At the same time, deliberately following healthy lifestyle principles can actually support your physical practice of Yoga. If you stop smoking, for example, your breathing will naturally expand and your circulation will improve. If you develop more positive qualities like openness, gentleness, and spirituality, I think you'll find that your experience of Yoga noticeably deepens. As with any lifestyle change, don't try to transform everything overnight. It's most important to proceed at a level and a pace that feels right to you.

As you strive toward an overall healthier lifestyle, keep the following goals in mind.

Have a Positive Intention

If negative thoughts can make you sick and tired, then positive thoughts can help make you well and happy. Because Yoga is a mind–body science, it acknowledges the importance of attitude and environment. It is so important to acknowledge something good in your life each day and experience gratitude. Be grateful that you are taking time for a Yoga therapy practice and taking control of your own healing process. Sometimes it helps to verbalize your positive thoughts or share happy or exciting ideas or events with others. Just to hear yourself talking this way can be beneficial. Words and thoughts are extremely powerful.

Exercise Faith and Prayer

Have you heard that faith is a powerful healer? Time and again people with strong faith have pulled themselves through difficult times or serious illnesses. Yoga teaches us to renew our faith in that which gives us sustenance. Whatever your religion or spiritual belief, now is the time to act on it, taking concrete steps to deepen and broaden your faith. To enhance your spirituality, you may want to practice some form of meditation. Chapter 5 offers some techniques.

Indulge Humor and Laughter

The late writer Norman Cousins helped cure himself from a chronic illness by the use of positive thoughts and humor. His approach? He rented his favorite Marx Brothers movies and laughed out loud watching them. Since the beginning of recorded history, laughter has been considered good medicine. Even if we can't laugh away serious problems, it may help us cope with them in a more positive way.

Take Time to Do What You Enjoy

Make time for activities that make you happy, bring you joy, and have a positive influence on you. Go for a walk, listen to music, spend time on a hobby, or visit with uplifting friends and relatives. Think about these things at the end of your practice, when your mind is quiet and focused, and you can see more clearly what is important and joyful to you.

For instance, many of the great Yoga masters recommend spending some quiet time in nature. Inspirational settings such as mountains, oceans, deserts, and lakes can recharge your batteries and rejuvenate your spirit. In fact, regular pilgrimages in nature are a vital part of many spiritual traditions. Making time for these activities can help improve your mental, emotional, and physical health, so it's important not to underestimate their importance.

Eat a Healthful Diet

Would you be surprised if I told you I am not a vegetarian? Most people I meet are amazed to learn that vegetarianism is not a prerequisite to learning or teaching Yoga. For seven out of my twenty years as a Yoga teacher and Yoga therapist, I tried to maintain some form of a vegetarian diet, including macrobiotic, vegan, and lacto-vegetarian. During those times, I never felt as good as I do when I include meat—mostly poultry and fish—in my regimen. I've come to the conclusion that everyone's constitution is different and we each have unique requirements.

While a vegetarian diet may not be appropriate for everyone, some health conditions benefit from skipping meat and dairy products altogether. Dean Ornish, M.D., with his pioneering research on heart disease, showed that a 10 percent fat, whole foods, vegetarian diet combined with aerobic exercise, stress management training, smoking cessation, and group support could reverse coronary artery disease. Because the program included more than just diet, it is hard to say that the decrease in heart conditions was due to the vegetarian diet. However, there is good evidence that lowering your cholesterol with a low-fat diet does decrease the risk of heart attack.

The nutritional suggestions that follow are not meant to replace any other diet information you may be pursuing. In fact, if you're interested in cleaning up your eating habits, I encourage you to speak with a well-trained nutritionist or health-care professional. Another option is to read some of the more credible nutrition books out there. (See the Resource Guide for our recommendations for excellent reference books on food and nutrition.)

When it comes to food, I know all too well how easy it is to read about the correct course to take but how hard it can be to shift your relationship with food and change your daily eating habits. Like so many people, I work hard to maintain my appropriate weight and have a tendency toward compulsive eating. This shocks people, because they often assume that a life committed to Yoga removes one from the common pitfalls and challenges of being human. I assure you it doesn't, and can prove it: My greatest adversaries are Ben and Jerry and their friend, Chunky Monkey.™

David Allen, a popular Los Angeles–based holistic medical doctor, recommends that patients ask themselves a critical question before every meal: "Is this what I would eat if my life depended on it?" He then quickly points out that it always does! With this advisory in mind, we offer the following guidelines for healthy eating:

* **Do not eat to the brim.** The Yoga approach for eating properly is to fill your stomach with half food, one quarter water, and one quarter air. This ensures you will leave the table satisfied but not too full, without that bloated feeling. (You should never have to loosen your belt to feel comfortable while or after eating.)

* **Eat in a relaxed, calm, and stress-free environment.** Avoid eating when you are upset, anxious, or rushed. Eliminate such distractions as TV, reading, and confrontational encounters.

* **Eat less.** As we get older, our metabolism tends to slow down, and we need fewer calories to maintain our health and weight. But learning to eat less cannot be accomplished by following the latest fad diet. It simply means that over time, you will benefit from slowly training yourself to choose smaller portions of healthier foods and to walk away when you're not quite full.

* **Chew well.** Efficient digestion is crucial to overall good health, and the digestive process starts in the mouth.

* **Fast a little bit each day.** The ancient Yoga philosophy suggested fasting for several days on end, which is not practical for our modern-day lifestyles. However, refraining from eating for three to four hours before you sleep is a healthy way to avoid heartburn, which can be uncomfortable and damage your esophagus and throat. You could also concentrate on fasting between meals—skipping the snacks in between (unless

your doctor recommends otherwise). You'll receive hunger signals when your body genuinely needs more nutrients, along with messages from your body about what nutrients it really needs. This helps you get in tune with your body, a crucial element of practicing Yoga.

* **Eat regularly and don't skip meals.** Eating a good healthy breakfast is a great way to start off your day, to enhance clear thinking and energize you for Yoga and other physical activities.

* **Go slowly.** After each bite or two, put your utensils down and ask yourself: Am I still hungry?

* **Choose a wide variety of foods.** Have at least five servings of fruits or vegetables every day as recommended by most nutritionists.

* **Emphasize whole foods and minimize prepackaged foods.** Try to avoid processed meats (such as sausage, bacon, and ham) as well as foods with additives and artificial ingredients, which can be detrimental to your health.

Just remember that with every step you take toward healthier eating habits, your Yoga practice will be enhanced. Whatever relief you're seeking, whatever physical, mental, and emotional changes you're after—they are likely to become reality much sooner if your food choices are consistent with good health practices.

Drink Plenty of Water

The human body is two thirds water. Obviously, we can't live or function properly without replenishing the water that we lose daily through our urinary tract (as urine), gastrointestinal system (as stool), respiratory system (as moisture in the air we breathe out), and our skin (sweating and evaporation). We take in water in the fluids we drink and the foods we eat to keep the water balanced in our bodies. Fortunately, almost all the foods we eat have significant water content, and most foods—plant and animal—are made of over 50 percent water. The kidney does a wonderful job of helping us keep that balance. When we drink more than we need, the kidney makes more urine. Conversely, when we don't take in enough fluids, the kidney holds on to more water. When this beautiful balanced system is working, our bodies are in a state of homeostasis.

Our job is to make sure we take in enough fluids to keep our bodies well hydrated and let the kidneys handle any extra fluid. Some nutritionists recommend a minimum of six to eight glasses of water daily. If you eat a lot of fruit, vegetables, soups, and other foods with high water content, then you may need fewer glasses of water or equivalent fluids such as juices and herb teas. If you sweat a lot while you exercise, you will need more fluids. Your body helps you keep this balance by giving you signals such as thirst and hunger and using the kidney to keep the homeostasis. Listen to your body's signals and make an effort to eat and drink healthy foods to maximize your health.

Many illnesses or injuries put our bodies at high risk of dehydration. This is especially true with high fevers, diarrhea, large burns, and vomiting. If you are suffering from any of these conditions, you should drink more fluids and get medical help when you are unable to replenish your losses to maintain your internal fluid balance.

Practice Breathing Exercises

In my twenty-year experience as a Yoga teacher and therapist, I have found that breathing exercises are the most profound healing tool Yoga has to offer—and also the simplest. Yoga breathing helps oxygenate the system, improve the musculature of the spine, strengthen the diaphragm, and relieve pain. It can energize you or calm you, whichever you need. You'll experience many benefits from taking quick five-minute Yoga breathing breaks whenever you need them during your day, especially if you're under stress (and who isn't?). Chapter 4 offers safe, time-tested Yoga breathing exercises and advanced techniques for building your energy.

Get Enough Rest

Perhaps one of the best-kept secrets for recovering and/or maintaining good health is proper rest and relaxation. When you don't get enough rest, you invite problems for any weak part of your system. In addition, the last thing you think about before sleep may be important. If you watch TV news just before you close your eyes, your mind may be filled with disturbing images, leading to less-than-restful sleep.

At bedtime try reading something pleasant or spiritual, listening to beautiful music, or just looking at photographs that give you a positive feeling. It's also an optimum time for reciting or writing a gratitude list.

Learn Meditation

One of the best ways to give yourself a relaxing break every day is to meditate. The ancients practiced Yoga postures, or *asanas* (Sanskrit for "seat"), to prepare themselves for many hours of sitting in meditation. The modern application of Yoga helps us counter the effects of our sedentary lifestyles and gives our minds a break from the constant distraction of media and the daily pressures that follow us wherever we go.

The mindful practice of Yoga is inherently meditative because it requires that you pay attention to the slow, subtle movements of your body from moment to moment. If you're not bringing your mind and body into harmony, you're just stretching or doing calisthenics, not practicing authentic Hatha Yoga.

The Yoga tradition also teaches a variety of meditation techniques that enhance the healing benefits of the physical postures. And in recent years, many Yoga teachers have incorporated methods from other traditions, especially Buddhism. Chapter 5 is devoted to meditations that complement the Yoga therapy in this book.

HOW YOGA THERAPY DIFFERS FROM YOGA

In 1989, when I co-founded the International Association of Yoga Therapists (IAYT), with Dr. Richard Miller, the name stirred controversy among our colleagues, because many established Yoga teachers contended that Yoga was by its very nature therapeutic. Why did we need a separate discipline called Yoga therapy? Since then, there has been ongoing dialogue in the Yoga community about what distinguishes Yoga therapy from ordinary Yoga. In a 2000 article in *International Journal of Yoga Therapy,* a panel of five well-known yoga experts attempts to define this developing discipline. Although no single definition has been widely adopted, the field of Yoga therapy has grown rapidly over the years, and the IAYT now boasts over a thousand members worldwide (see the Resource Guide).

In my own view, Yoga therapy adapts the practices of Yoga to the needs of people with specific or persistent health problems. Frequently, these people can't attend group Yoga classes and need one-on-one attention. Yoga therapy can serve as a transition into group Yoga classes, as it did for my friend Chris. I first met Chris years ago when we both attended El Camino College in Torrance, California. Her sorority and my fraternity often did fun things together. One night at a party, Chris had a severe asthma attack. We all gathered around, very alarmed, as she struggled to catch her breath. We rushed her to the emergency room, and, with treatment, she recovered. But I never forgot the experience.

After college we lost touch with one another. Then, twenty-five years later, I bumped into Chris while on my way to teach a Yoga class in Malibu. Surprised and delighted, we reminisced about old times, and I asked about her asthma. Apparently she had been using various medications and taking allergy shots ever since the attack in college. Occasionally, she still woke up wheezing and ended up in the hospital. Her asthma could also be triggered by the slightest aerobic exercise. I immediately recommended Yoga therapy.

After a few private lessons, in which she learned breathing exercises similar to those recommended for asthma in Chapter 8, she was able to begin Yoga practice at home on her own. She also began taking Chinese herbs, and a few weeks later she joined my twice-a-week group class. After three months of regular classes, herbs, and Yoga breathing exercises, her asthma resolved and Chris stopped taking her medication and allergy shots completely. For the past eight years, she has been a regular in my Malibu class and she has been asthma- and medication-free the whole time, occasionally using an inhaler for allergies.

Like Chris, many people benefit very quickly from a Yoga program designed for their specific ailments, which is what we offer in Part III of this book. But ordinary Yoga practice can also have a therapeutic effect. I learned this from my own experience, when my chronic back pain gradually disappeared as I continued to attend a regular Hatha Yoga class. However, if I had been able to get one-on-one Yoga therapy specific to my back pain, I'm sure my healing would have occurred more quickly.

Both Yoga and Yoga therapy need to be adapted to the culture in which they are taught. The postures and procedures recommended at a traditional Yoga therapy center in India, for example, aren't necessarily appropriate for students in the United States. Because Yoga therapists may work in concert with physicians and other conventional health-care providers, we need to use language and procedures that they can understand. When I communicate with medical providers, I explain that Yoga therapy is the practical application of Yoga principles for people with special physical, emotional, or spiritual needs or challenges. In the rest of the book, I will show you how to use the time-honored practices of Yoga therapy to significantly improve your health and well-being.

2

How You Can Benefit from

Yoga Therapy

When you're relaxed and free of stress and your mind is focused and calm, your body has an innate capacity to heal itself. Your natural state is one of balance, and it is only when a negative external force intervenes that you become out of balance—you experience ill health. Your practice of Yoga encourages health by reducing stress, enhancing concentration, increasing feelings of comfort and ease, and helping bring your whole being back into harmony and balance.

Physically, the postures of Hatha Yoga promote balance by equally stretching the right and left sides and the front and back parts of your body. This symmetrical approach gradually corrects any tendency you might have to favor one side or part over another. On a muscular level, Yoga helps you achieve balance by both stretching and strengthening the muscles throughout your body. Muscles that are loose and well stretched are less likely to be injured, much like taffy that when cold can be snapped, but when warm is pliable and gives.

But the deeper balance that Yoga affords comes from the combination of concentration, stress reduction, and relaxation it teaches. When you're focused in the present, free of stress about past or future, relaxed, alert, and feeling contented or even joyful, your body tends to perform at optimal levels and naturally gravitates toward a state of optimal health.

If you own a computer, you know how frustrating it can be when the machine freezes up, especially when you're hurrying to meet a deadline. Often, it seems, computers crash when they're running several programs and handling too much information at once. Usually the only solution is to turn off the machine and give it a rest. When you turn it back on, it does some checking and adjusting of systems, everything falls back into place, and you can get back to work.

In the same way, your body and mind can become overworked and out of whack; they can even "crash" and become injured or ill. Yoga provides the break your mind–body needs to avoid crashes, helping you stay in balance and function at your highest level. In this chapter, we'll take a closer look at the many unique benefits of Yoga and Yoga therapy.

STRESS REDUCTION

With the explosion in the past decade of new devices that speed the flow of information, I've watched in alarm as people's stress levels have risen accordingly. From the moment we grab our coffee and begin making phone calls in the morning, to the final checking of e-mail before going to bed at night, we're barraged with a seemingly endless stream of complex challenges that we feel increasingly hard pressed to meet. As our minds speed to keep up, our bodies tense and contract in response. The result can be extraordinary levels of stress, which may at times threaten to spin out of control.

Though stress levels may be higher than ever, the experience of stress is as old as humankind. In fact, it's hard wired into our DNA in what psychologists call the "fight-or-flight" response. Imagine one of our primitive ancestors coming out of a cave and confronting a saber-toothed tiger eye to eye. He would be scared to death. Adrenaline would start pumping into his bloodstream, his heart rate and breathing would accelerate to speed the circulation of oxygen and nutrients, his muscles would tighten, and his eyes would widen to increase his visual acuity. At this point, his body would be ready for the physical exertion of a battle or a fast run. Until he took action, his body would experience acute stress; once he responded, however, his stress would rapidly diminish, as he naturally channeled his energy into movement.

Unfortunately, the challenges that most of us face today don't require, or even allow, the vigorous physical activity for which the stress response prepares us. When you are faced with a deadline, have an argument with your spouse, receive a stressful series of phone calls, or are put on the spot during a meeting, you are unable to strike back or flee. Instead, you remain frozen in place with no physical way to express anger or fear. As a result, your muscles remain tense and contracted—unless and until you deliberately stretch them.

Recently I had an opportunity to experience the fight-or-flight response first-hand. Fortunately, my years of Yoga practice allowed me to defuse my stress rapidly—and neutralize a potentially inflammatory situation, as well. Kaustub Desi-kachar, the son of my Yoga teacher, had come to visit with his new wife, and I was giving them a scenic tour of Los Angeles. As we were driving through the hills, a gang of bikers rode up behind us, revving their engines. They seemed annoyed that we were going the speed limit and blocking their way. Afraid of what they might do and concerned for the safety of my special passengers, I found my emotions going into overdrive, with my heart pounding and my adrenaline surging. Drawing on my Yoga experience, I took several long deep breaths and relaxed my body as much as I could.

Finally, the lead biker pulled up beside us and made an obscene gesture using one of his fingers (you can guess which one). I smiled and showed him a couple fingers of my own—the peace sign. Surprised, he hesitated for a moment, then smiled back, shook his head, and returned to his gang. With a few breaths I had reduced my stress and brought a resolution to our encounter.

Even though I had been able to respond without aggression, my muscles held the physical memory of stress and tension until I could physically stretch them later with Yoga. The body holds muscle length constant the way a thermostat holds a temperature constant in a house. Muscles get set to a certain shortness and cannot lengthen on their own; they must be pulled by an outside force, such as a Yoga stretch. If you stretch consciously and deliberately, your brain is encouraged to reset your muscles to a new, more relaxed length. Your muscles are less likely to tear and are more efficient. Your mind–body returns to a state of balance.

Many Yoga practices counter the fight-or-flight response and invite the body to move in the opposite direction toward peace and calm. Gentle stretching lengthens your muscles, reducing physical tension. Yoga breathing slows your respiration. Inverted postures can help lower your blood pressure by decreasing your heart rate, relaxing your arteries, and reducing levels of the stress hormone noradrenaline. Resting Yoga postures allow you to let go of physical and mental effort. Meditative practices help you put fear and anger into perspective. With increased calm and relaxation comes a decrease in your level of cortisol, an adrenal hormone that inhibits immune system function. This keeps your body at optimal alert against disease.

IMPROVED CIRCULATION

When the circulation of blood is restricted in any way, the cells of your body may not get the oxygen and nutrients they need to function effectively. As a result, your energy may plummet, your mood and mental capacities may suffer, and ultimately your overall health may be impaired. Good circulation is a prerequisite for good health.

The practice of Yoga improves the flow of blood to and from the heart in a number of significant ways. Standing Yoga postures squeeze the veins in the leg and gently push blood back toward the heart, similar to other exercises, such as walking, that contract the leg muscles. Yoga postures that lift the legs above the heart use the force of gravity to do much the same thing.

When you practice a variety of Yoga poses, you systematically position your arms, legs, trunk, and head both higher and lower than your heart, draining, then refreshing the blood supply to each area, improving the delivery of oxygen and nutrients, and removing carbon dioxide and waste products. In addition, when you practice twisting and bending postures, you compress certain muscles and organs and release them. This action squeezes the blood from the area and allows fresh blood to enter, much as you might squeeze and then soak a sponge. Fatigue is reduced; every part of your body receives its proper nutrient supply.

INCREASED FLEXIBILITY AND STRENGTH

In almost any Yoga pose, especially the standing postures that work against gravity, you are both stretching and strengthening your muscles. For example, when you stand and bend forward from your hip joints, the pelvis tilts on the tops of the thigh bones and lengthens the hamstring muscles on the backs of your thighs, which run from your sit bones down to the backs of your knees. When you come up out of the standing forward bend, you lift up your body weight by contracting (and thereby strengthening) the same muscles you stretched on the way down.

This combination of stretching and strengthening makes Yoga an especially good routine for professional athletes, who need to maximize their flexibility to avoid costly injuries. Many athletes have discovered the benefits of Yoga in recent years, including the 2000, 2001, and 2002 World Champion Los Angeles Lakers, who practiced Yoga weekly on their way to the championship. Former Laker center Kareem Abdul Jabbar was a devoted practitioner of Yoga and meditated before every game to reduce stress. He set National Basketball Association (NBA) records for scoring the most points in a career, winning the greatest number of Most Valuable Player (MVP) awards, playing in the most All-Star games, and being the oldest active player. I always wonder how much his Yoga practice contributed to his greatness.

ENHANCED CONCENTRATION

By demanding your singular attention to the present moment, Yoga trains you to concentrate and clear your mind of distracting thoughts and preoccupations. If you don't give your full attention while doing a physical posture, you're liable to hurt yourself. Yoga demands that you listen to the voice within, your own unique body wisdom, to go to your limit without unwisely exceeding it. Even just attempting to hold a simple pose requires concentration. If you're balancing on one foot, you have to concentrate or you will fall right over.

Paying close attention to your sensations in each pose tends to clear whatever else is on your mind at the moment. This is meditation. To the extent you are focused on your breath and body, you are not having thoughts about business or personal matters. That part of your mind is quiet. By the time you get to the end of your routine, your mind is focused and calm and your body, relaxed. Ultimately, the concentration acquired from the physical practice of Yoga spills over to other areas of your life.

Students who practice Yoga regularly tell me that they find it much easier to become engrossed in their work and to remain undistracted for extended periods. They also report that their intimate relationships improve because they can stay present and available to partners and friends far more readily than before.

OVERALL SENSE OF WELL-BEING

In 1989 I founded the corporate Yoga program at the J. Paul Getty Museum in Malibu, California. The classes were held at lunchtime in the museum's boardroom and attracted students from many levels of the corporate hierarchy. Just outside the boardroom was a guard station that most of the students passed on their way to and from class. After I had been offering the program for three months, one of the security guards working the booth gave me a memorable compliment. He said, "Since you've been teaching Yoga classes here, everyone that passes my station is so much nicer to me. They tell me they feel happier after your class."

According to ancient philosophy, Yoga postures open spaces throughout the body that allow the life force (prana) to circulate more freely. Certain poses seem to create space between the vertebrae, within the joints, and around the internal organs; other poses feel like they lift the heart and open space between the neck and shoulders. Many approaches to alternative medicine maintain that disease and pain are caused, in part, by "stuck" energy. Constricted or blocked channels where nervous energy, air, or blood do not flow properly lead to trouble. By improving circulation and reducing muscle tension, most people who practice Yoga find that they gain more energy from the process.

Exactly why Yoga affords most people who practice it an amplified sense of well-being is not yet completely understood by science. We do know that Yoga has numerous benefits, both physical and psychological. In my experience with students, I've found that when individuals reduce their stress, relax their muscles, and calm their mind, they report more enjoyment in simply being alive.

This is important because, unfortunately, not every ailment can be healed. In some cases, the practice of Yoga works not to eliminate a disorder completely, but to minimize its physical, mental, and emotional impact. A Yoga lifestyle can help heal your heart and mind, bringing you to a state of peace and well-being. This is where the true joy of living comes from, and you can have it even if you're living with chronic illness or disability.

Take a moment to imagine that you have achieved a state of optimum health and balance on every level: physical, emotional, and spiritual. Imagine those migraines dwindling, that depression lifting, that hay fever subsiding. What would your life be like? How would you feel? Certainly your stress level would diminish, and your work and relationships would improve. More important, you might even experience an inner peace and a radiant vitality that external circumstances could not easily disturb.

Yoga is a powerful tool that can help you approach this state of optimum health, harmony, and well-being. We're confident that Yoga therapy can improve your health in significant ways, whatever your present condition may happen to be.

3

Getting Started with

Yoga Therapy

Some of the traditional Yoga schools in India still recommend principles and practices that would seem quite strange and distasteful to us Westerners. On my first trip to India, I had the opportunity to visit a number of Yoga therapy clinics. My first stumbling block was that Yoga therapy practice was always recommended at sunrise (5:30 A.M.). My next challenge came when I reported a digestive problem. I was instructed to drink ten glasses of salt water, which was followed by numerous regurgitations. As unpleasant as it was, it actually did make me feel better. I was closely supervised by an expert and had plenty of time to rest afterward. However, because this could be quite dangerous, we do not recommend this therapy under any circumstances. I mention it as an illustration of how the principles of Yoga practice vary from culture to culture.

In the West, a Yoga therapy practice has to be compatible with our culture as well as practical, user friendly, and safe. There are several important principles that I feel capture the essentials of an effective Yoga therapy practice for our modern world. They include the following:

- Commitment to a daily Yoga therapy program
- Combining breath with movement
- Emphasizing function over form
- Incorporating dynamic and static principles of motion
- Focusing on the spine
- Slowing down your pace
- Avoiding competition
- Staying faithful to sequencing

KEEP YOUR VOWS OF COMMITMENT

This book is designed to be a do-it-yourself program. However, I want to be right up front about the fact that it takes terrific discipline to practice Yoga faithfully and regularly on your own. Knowing this, you may want to consciously commit yourself to doing some form of practice every day, even if it's only for three minutes.

Choose a comfortable place and time in which you can practice consistently each day. It can be any place that gives you enough space and preferably some peace and quiet. It is okay to practice after a small meal or snack, but you need to wait two to three hours after a heavy meal. Once you have begun your daily practice, be patient and compassionate with yourself. Yoga will get easier each time you do it, and eventually you will build up the momentum for a longer practice. Realize it may take a month or more for your daily Yoga to become a habit. If you persevere even when you'd rather quit, Yoga will help you feel better each day, and pretty soon you will not feel complete without it.

EMPOWER YOUR MOVEMENT
WITH BREATH

Chapter 4 outlines the reasons and techniques for Yoga breathing. It is essential that Yoga breathing accompany movement at all times. Always move slowly and keep your mind focused on the breath coupled with movement. Coordinating breath and movement supports the union of the body, breath, and mind. Focusing on breathing helps you concentrate on what you are doing in that very moment, rather than thinking about your car payment or what you're going to have for dinner.

As a basic rule, inhale when the Yoga posture opens the body, exhale when the position folds the body. For example, if you are executing a standing forward bend (which is like a toe touch), inhale as you lift your arms up, and exhale as you are folding or bending forward and down.

There are four ways that your body moves naturally with the breath: Forward bend (flexion), back bend (extension), side bend (lateral flexion), and twist (rotation).

- Exhale as you are going into a forward bend, side bend, or twist. Inhale as you are coming out.
- Inhale as you are going into a back bend, and exhale as you are coming out.

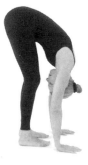

EXHALE

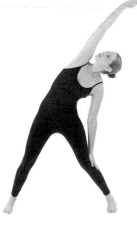

EXHALE

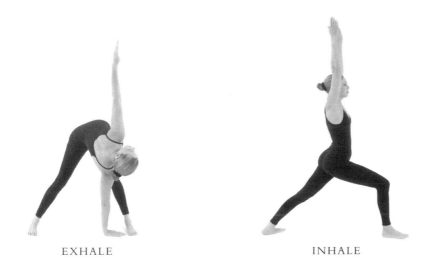

EXHALE   INHALE

If you are in the middle of a breath and movement cycle and you run out of breath before you have completed the movement, pause your movement briefly and then return back to the starting place. For example, if you are raising your arms on an inhalation and run out of breath before they are fully extended, just stop your arms where they are and lower them on the exhalation. Let the length of your breath determine how far you move into the posture. Eventually your breath will deepen, and you will be able to complete the full breath and movement cycle. Sometimes you hold or stay in a posture for several breaths. When you do, it is okay to increase the stretch on each succeeding breath.

EMPHASIZE FUNCTION
OVER FORM

Many Yoga books illustrate a standing forward bend with the model's forehead touching her knees, her legs and arms straight, and the palms of her hands on the ground. While the form in this posture looks great, the truth is only about 10 percent of the entire population can achieve it, and it's not necessary for a successful Yoga practice.

Although some practitioners might disagree, there is no perfect Yoga posture; what matters most in Yoga therapy is the function, not the form. You should never try to force yourself into an ideal posture. While maintaining good technique, don't try to push yourself too far. One of the tools you can use to achieve the function of the pose is a concept I call "forgiving limbs."

For example, if you're trying to do a standing forward bend, your legs and back may be stiff and hamstrings tight. As you move into position and feel a pull in the back of your legs, be forgiving. Bend your knees enough to fit your needs. Softening your legs will bring more freedom to the lower back. Softening your arms will bring more freedom to your upper back, neck, and shoulders. As you become more flexible you can begin to straighten your legs, but do not lock or hyperextend any of your limbs. The primary function of the standing forward bend is to stretch your back, with a secondary goal of loosening up your hamstrings. This principle also applies to standing side bends and twists.

You'll be amazed at how your body instinctively knows what to do. Relax, tune in, and follow your inner guide. Note that the models shown on page 25 have soft limbs.

USE THE DYNAMIC AND THE STATIC

When we are moving in and out of postures, we are using the *dynamic*. When we are holding a posture, we are using the *static*. Yoga practice is most effective if we incorporate both the dynamic and the static into our routines. We do this by slowly moving in and out of most Yoga postures a few times before holding them. There are exceptions: in some postures we use either the dynamic or the static, but not both. Your Yoga routine as a whole will incorporate the two principles.

There are distinct advantages to the combination dynamic–static approach. First, using movement before holding each posture provides a safety factor by enhancing the circulation (or blood flow) in the area and thus preparing the muscles and joints for the holding phase. Moving in and out of postures before holding them allows for a deeper stretch. This concept is a variation of what is called proprioceptive neuromuscular facilitation (PNF). In a nutshell, if you tighten a muscle just before you stretch it, it will stretch farther. (It's like bending your knees before jumping rather than jumping from a standing position.) This is especially true for many of the standing postures in which you are bending forward and stretching the major muscles with gravity, then rising up against gravity and tightening the same muscles.

For many postures, we recommend that before you hold them, you move in and out at least three times, but not more than six. Hold a posture for six to eight breaths, or roughly thirty seconds. Continue your Yoga breathing while holding. Do not hold your breath.

For each Yoga posture suggested in this book, the number of repetitions and/or the holding time are specified. Follow the instructions carefully, noting that a few postures incorporate repetition without holding, and others instruct you to hold but not repeat. After practicing a while, you'll get a feel for it. Your practice may vary, depending on how you are feeling on any given day.

Don't worry if your limbs tremble from time to time while holding a pose. That's a normal reaction in the beginning, until you build strength and become familiar with the routines. If the trembling begins to feel like an earthquake, then ease out of the pose gently.

Though you may be tempted to bounce while holding certain Yoga positions—don't. Bouncing can lead to a distracted focus or even an injury. The danger of bouncing can be compared to hopping on a balance beam as opposed to just walking. The chances of slipping and injuring yourself are much greater.

Some of the postures in this book contain specific instructions for coming out of them, because it is important that you do it a certain way. If the posture does not have these instructions, just move your body gently to the starting position for the next pose.

FOCUS ON THE SPINE

There is an old saying: You are as old as your spine. Conversely, you are as young as your spine is flexible. I believe this to be true. The next time you're in a large group, observe how some people seem older than their years because they have become so stiff in the spine.

The longer we are on this planet, the more opportunity gravity has to create a negative effect on our bodies, including compressing the spine. Yoga postures offer a method for decompressing the spine, creating a feeling of space between the vertebrae, resulting in enhanced postural alignment. This can reduce stress to the musculoskeletal, digestive, respiratory, and circulatory systems. It is why so many of the principles of practice support the concept of focusing on the spine. Function over form, forgiving limbs, and dynamic and static movements are all principles that yield more freedom to the spine. For best results, your Yoga movements should feel fluid, as though your joints are moving through water.

KEEP IT SLOW

No matter how brief your Yoga routine may be on any given day, Yoga should never be done in a hurry. The whole idea of Yoga is to slow down and quiet the multitudinous distractions of the mind.

In many parts of our lives, we are rewarded by speed of accomplishment. Yoga takes that rule and turns it upside down. The more slowly you go in Yoga, the greater your rewards will be.

Do not rush through postures, and remember that resting poses are as important as active ones. Warming up is as crucial as cooling down, and always remember the tiny pauses between each inhale and exhale.

Your eyes can be open or closed during Yoga practice, but closing the eyes helps some people to slow down. Choose whichever is most comfortable for you each time you practice. Usually, standing or balancing poses require the eyes to be open, while resting and restorative poses can be enjoyed more fully with the eyes shut.

FORGET ABOUT COMPETITION

Yoga is not a competition—not even with yourself. Yoga encourages you to move at your own pace and not judge yourself. I've been doing Yoga for more than twenty years, and sometimes I practice like a beginner when I'm recovering from an injury or just plain exhausted.

Your physical condition is affected by so many factors that are constantly in flux: hormones, hydration, mind-set, stress, activity levels, and emotions. Every day your body will feel different, especially if you've been ill or are dealing with a chronic ailment.

It's easy to say and hard to do, but suspend all judgments when it comes to your Yoga performance. It's not about how difficult the posture is or how long you hold it. The beauty of your practice is that you will receive benefits, even if you're doing only conservative postures and holding them for only a short period of time.

Ancient Yoga teachings say that where your mind goes, your circulation goes. Visualize the bodily area you are working on, and if you notice tension or resistance, visualize your breath going to the area to soothe it and smooth it out. This does not mean breathe into the pain. There is no gain from pain in Yoga. Listen to your body. Stay tuned in with a dialogue, not a monologue. Your motto should be: Challenge myself, don't strain myself.

ALWAYS USE PROPER SEQUENCING

There is logic to the sequence of the postures in each of this book's routines. The art of sequencing involves placing the postures in a specific order to maximize the benefits. A good Yoga therapy program has an intelligent plan that takes into consideration your ultimate goal, the safest and most efficient way to accomplish that goal, your skill level, and the amount of time allotted for practice.

The routines in this book are designed with the assumption that you are new to Yoga and that you are busy and have limited time to devote to it. Each routine has a specific goal, either general conditioning or managing an ailment. Ranging in length from ten to thirty minutes, they are short enough to fit your lifestyle yet long enough to be effective.

The routines are safe, proven, and always start with a transition posture that leads you gently from your hectic day into your routine with Yoga breathing. Next, a warmup prepares the body, followed by the main postures, which are selected to address the goal. Compensation postures bring your body back into neutral. Finally, breathing exercises and relaxation techniques allow you to rest before you move on to your next activity. Because Yoga therapy routines are so carefully designed to be safe and effective, it is important you do the postures in the order recommended.

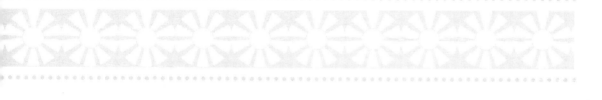

PART II

Putting Yoga Therapy

into Action

Now that you've read Part I, you have all the background you need to begin using your body, breath, and mind to practice Yoga therapy techniques. The next three chapters will instruct you in basic Yoga breathing, relaxation, meditation, and postures. They will get you acclimated to Yoga and prepare you for the ailment-specific routines presented in Part III. So grab a towel and some comfortable clothes, and let's get to work!

4

The Wind in Your Sails:

Yoga Breathing

Last year, my friend Merry traveled cross-country to attend her father's funeral. Upon arrival, she was exhausted, emotionally distressed, and nervous. Her hands were shaking, and she could feel her heart racing; but she was determined to deliver a eulogy at the service. Just before addressing the crowd, she went into a quiet room and practiced five minutes of a simple Yoga technique called Focused Breathing (page 39). Her hands stopped shaking and she felt her pulse returning to normal. She was centered and tranquil, able to read a tribute beautifully without her voice so much as cracking. It was a remarkable illustration of just how calming the breath can be.

The breath is the most important tool in Yoga. Even when you cannot move your body—you're stuck in that big business meeting or that tiny airplane seat— you can still practice Yoga with your breath. Yoga breathing is simply using various techniques to breathe in a slow and focused manner, allowing you to concentrate on your breath and become more conscious of your body's rhythms.

The ability to affect your body's functioning through the way you breathe is recognized in many areas of modern life. When you're angry and tempted to explode verbally, you're advised to "take a deep breath." People who are experiencing acute or chronic pain are often taught specialized breathing techniques as a way of managing their pain: Women in labor use variations on Lamaze breathing; and other pain sufferers, such as those with cancer or fibromyalgia, are taught deep breathing exercises to reduce their need for narcotics. Biofeedback has been around for decades and includes instruction in deep breathing to help control physiological reactions that are ordinarily unconscious, such as heart rate and blood pressure. The martial arts use the breath as a means of keeping the body, mind, and emotions in control. Even athletes, such as Olympic swimmers and marathon runners, must consciously work on their breathing techniques to improve their physical and mental functioning.

Your body's breathing center is actually in the brainstem, where many of your autonomic functions are controlled, such as your heart rate, blood pressure, skin temperature, and digestive process. Breathing is the only autonomic function that you can control at will, kind of like a manual override. Research indicates that when you manually take control of your breathing, you are given a little bit of control over your other autonomic functions as well. Thus deep, measured Yoga breathing affects the respiratory system by increasing absorption of oxygen and release of carbon dioxide. It can calm a rapid heart rate and relax muscle tension. Yoga breathing also helps strengthen abdominal muscles and improve posture.

Probably the two most important benefits of Yoga breathing are its effectiveness in stress reduction and pain management. Since stress is an underlying factor exacerbating virtually all other health conditions, the reduction of stress through regular Yoga breathing can have a major effect on your health. Yoga breathing reduces stress by curbing the flow of adrenaline and other stress hormones. It also quiets the distractions of the mind and signals the brain to minimize perception of pain. I have witnessed literally hundreds of my clients over the years reduce or totally eliminate acute symptoms of back pain using Belly Breathing, a Yoga technique explained later in this chapter. The most phenomenal aspect of Yoga breathing is that you are in control. You can send health-enhancing Yoga breathing messages to your body any time, anywhere.

Entire textbooks have been written about the physiology of breathing; but don't worry, we're not going to go into that much detail here. To understand the Yoga approach, you need to know only a few basic things about breathing.

When you think of your breath, you might immediately think of the lungs, but the lungs are actually passive organs that hitch along on the breathing ride. The real force behind breathing is the respiratory musculature, driven by the diaphragm. It has been said that the diaphragm is responsible for about 75 percent of the effort of quiet breathing. I wonder how many folks have any idea where their diaphragm is or how it works.

Diaphragm literally means "partition," aptly enough, since it divides the thorax (rib cage) above from the abdomen below. You could say that the diaphragm is the floor of the former and the roof of the latter. The lungs and heart sit right on top of the diaphragm, and the stomach and liver nestle right below it. Our diaphragm's rhythms—powered by our breathing—affect these organs, partially explaining how breathing influences so many other functions of the body.

THE DIAPHRAGM

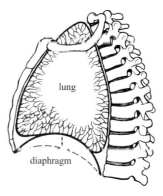

The circumference of the diaphragm attaches to the lower rim of the rib cage, which makes it look in outline like a giant kidney bean. It also has two long skinny muscular attachments, called crura, along the sides of the lumbar vertebrae. They always remind me of a long pair of pigtails.

Each inhale is initiated when the diaphragm contracts and descends. The double dome flattens out and pushes down (only about an inch) against the abdominal contents, which have nowhere to go but out. I'm sure you have noticed how your belly puffs every time you inhale. That puffing, which allows the easy descent of the diaphragm, is made possible by the relaxation of the rectus abdominis, a muscle that runs in a flat sheet between your pubic bone below and the bottom of the sternum above.

The contraction and descent of the diaphragm (assisted by a few sidekick respiratory muscles) increases the volume of the thorax, lowering its pressure relative to the outside world. Just like wind is caused by air flowing from areas of high pressure to areas of low pressure, fresh air from the outside rushes into the thorax, and voilà!—you inhale. Then on the exhale, this whole thing gets reversed. The diaphragm slowly relaxes and returns to its dome shape, egged on by the contraction of the rectus, which pushes back and up against the abdominal contents. This decreases the volume of the thorax and the inhaled air, now full of carbon dioxide and other waste stuff we no longer need, is forced out of the lungs. Whew!

If all of this information makes you a little breathless, just remember that the diaphragm is essentially a pump. Like a piston inside a cylinder it moves up and down, sucking air in and squeezing it out of our lungs.

THE YOGA PERSPECTIVE ON BREATHING

In the ancient Sanskrit language, the word for *breath* is the same as the word for *life, prana*. From the Yoga point of view, the air that we breathe contains more than just oxygen, carbon dioxide, and other gases; it contains prana, our life force, that substance from which all life and activity is derived. Prana enters our bodies when we are born and mysteriously leaves us when we die. In the same way that the concept of a person's soul is unlikely to be proven by modern science, so the idea of prana remains unproven. Yet modern science does acknowledge oxygen itself as the most basic of human needs, and the advanced Yoga breathing techniques called prana-yama (prah-nah-YAM-a) teach us to make maximum use of our oxygen for optimum health and vitality. The principle of a life force energy is common in various cultures; in China it is known as Chi, in Japan as Ki.

Just as oxygen is stored and circulated in the blood, Yoga literature suggests that prana is stored and circulated in our bodies. Ancient Yogis practiced Yoga breathing to maintain their prana and thereby increase their health and vitality. Whether or not you accept the concept of prana, Yoga breathing's physiology and benefits are well documented in contemporary science, with advantages ranging from decreased stress to improved mental focus to deeper relaxation.

YOGA BREATHING TECHNIQUES

Think of a sailboat, cutting swiftly through a sun-glinted sea—sails unfurled, bow slightly bobbing—a beautiful sight! Its sleek design conceals the powerful framework and the elaborate systems that all interact for smooth sailing. But without the magic ingredient—wind—these systems are useless. Similarly, without breath, all of the elaborate systems of our bodies would be useless. Just as there are different types of wind to propel a sailboat, some more desirable than others, there are different types of breathing available to us, some more healthy for our bodies than others and each having its own unique effect.

When you're out on that sailboat and the wind comes in short, unpredictable gusts from a variety of directions, you'll have difficulty controlling the craft, and you're going to be tossed around. However, with a calm, steady yet persistent breeze, all systems work in effortless harmony for a pleasant ride. Yoga breathing can bring our bodies into this harmonious state of smooth sailing.

The idea behind Yoga breathing is to make a change in your mental and physical demeanor. It modifies how you normally breathe to a slower, more conscious, focused, and complete breath. It also helps tone and strengthen your abdomen. From the Yoga point of view, the abdomen is your body's center of movement, and if the abdomen is flabby there is a greater tendency toward ill health. Most of the Yoga breathing techniques in this chapter emphasize gently drawing the belly in during exhalation to strengthen and tone those muscles.

There is an old Yoga axiom, The nose was meant for breathing and the mouth was meant for eating. With few exceptions, Yoga breathing is classically taught through the nose, both on inhalation and on exhalation. There is both ageless wisdom and scientific knowledge to support this concept of nasal breathing. First, when you breathe through the nose it slows the breath down because the air is moving through two small openings instead of the one big opening in your mouth. Next, when you breathe through the nose, the air is filtered and warmed (for more on why this is healthy, see Chapter 8). In more advanced breathing techniques of pranayama, the nostrils are opened and closed using the fingertips—referred to as digital pranayama—which affects the length and quality of the breath. Keep in mind that Yoga breathing has its time and place; other forms of exercise, such as swimming and jogging, require different kinds of breathing.

There are temporary conditions, such as seasonal allergies, and permanent conditions, such as a deviated septum, that can make nasal breathing difficult. However, most people with nasal allergies or a deviated septum will be able to do Yoga breathing with no problems. If you have difficulty with nasal breathing, consult a doctor. You may also try to choose positions that keep your body upright and try to determine what part of the day is best for you to do Yoga. If medical care and these suggestions do not work to improve your nasal breathing, try inhaling with your nose, exhaling with your mouth. As a last resort, go ahead and use your mouth for breathing.

When practicing these breathing techniques, it's normal to feel a little lightheaded. Since you are breathing abnormally you could, at first, feel dizzy or a little spacey. Not to worry—it's normal. If this happens to you, just rest for a few minutes. These symptoms will be replaced by a greater sense of well-being.

How to Combine Breath and Movement for Yoga

To achieve the optimum benefits from Yoga, your movement should always be contained within a cycle of breath. You begin your breath, then begin your movement. Complete the movement, then complete the breath. A simple bar graph illustrates the relationship of breath and movement:

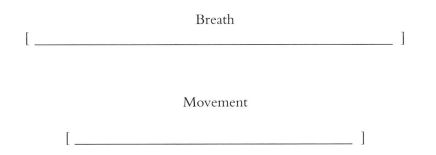

Another way to consider the relationship between breath and movement is to think about your breath as a wave in the ocean, and the movement as the surfer. The surfer waits for the wave to begin, rides it, then finishes the ride before the wave ends. While practicing Yoga, you first start the wave of your breath, then begin and end your movement, then let the wave subside.

BASIC YOGA BREATHING

Yoga Breathing Techniques

The following techniques can be used for any of the recommended Yoga routines in this book or as separate exercises while lying or sitting.

If you are using any of the breathing techniques as part of a Yoga routine from Part III, follow those instructions for the number of repetitions. If you are using a breathing technique as a separate exercise, repeat a minimum of twenty to thirty times.

First we'll explore four simple Yoga breathing techniques: Focused Breathing, Belly Breathing, Belly-to-Chest Breathing, and Chest-to-Belly Breathing.

Focused Breathing

The easiest way for beginners to get started with Yoga breathing is to use Focused Breathing. It will help you practice the basic elements common in the more advanced techniques. Think of focused breathing as training wheels for complete Yoga breathing.

Part One

1. Sit comfortably in a chair and place your hands on your thighs. Your palms can face up or down.
2. Bring your back up nice and tall and close your eyes.
3. Observe your state of mind and natural resting breath for a few cycles. Then consciously begin to make your inhalation and exhalation longer, smoother, and deeper than normal. Take control of your breath, rather than letting it happen on its own. Breathe through your nose.
4. Let there be a natural pause at the top of the inhalation as well as after the exhalation. Notice the effect the pause has on your state of mind. The pause is to help lengthen the breath and to remind you to slow down and concentrate on

the process of breath. This pause is an introduction to meditation, the first step toward quieting the mind.

5. Notice how your breath moves your body, especially your rib cage and shoulders. When you inhale the body expands; when you exhale the body contracts.

6. Focus mentally on just your Yoga breathing. When your mind drifts away, bring it back to the breath. Listen to the sound your breath makes. Feel the air entering your nose and expanding your lungs. This is how the breath is used to connect the body and the mind. Eventually the breath and movement become a form of meditation. When you practice focusing, you'll soon notice improved concentration and the quieting of your mind, which is one of the ultimate goals of Yoga. As your concentration improves in Yoga, it also improves in other aspects of your life.

7. After 25 rounds of Focused Breathing, gradually let your breath come back to normal and sit for a few minutes with your eyes closed. Think about your state of mind when you first started and then compare it to how you now feel. You'll be amazed at how you can shift your overall energy with just your breath.

Part Two

When you're familiar with Part One, begin to gently draw the belly in as you exhale. Make sure you don't strain yourself or pull the belly in too much. Sometimes it helps to visualize wearing a belt with a large buckle in front. During the exhalation phase gently pull the belly in away from the buckle.

Belly Breathing

Belly Breathing is often used in Yoga for relaxation and pain relief. It differs from Part Two of Focused Breathing in that it requires focus on the belly in both the inhalation and the exhalation phases.

1. Imagine that you are wearing a wide elastic band around your waist. When you inhale, expand the belly and the band in all directions—front, sides, and back.
2. During exhalation contract the abdomen. Pause after both the inhalation and the exhalation, and try to keep the chest as still as possible.
3. Repeat 20 to 30 times if you're doing the breathing exercise without movement or as directed in your Yoga therapy routine.

Belly-to-Chest Breathing

Belly-to-Chest Breathing is often referred to as classic or three-part breathing. It was popularized by Indian Yoga teachers who came to America in the 1960s. This technique incorporates a wave-like motion involving the belly, ribs, and chest and is great for giving your body a little oxygen lift. You can use this breathing where indicated in the Yoga therapy routines or when you feel your brain needs a jump-start to help you focus.

1. As you inhale, expand your belly, then your ribs, and finally your chest. Pause.
2. As you exhale, release your chest and ribs, then contract your belly. Pause.
3. Repeat 20 to 30 times if you're doing the breathing exercise without movement or as directed in your Yoga therapy routine.

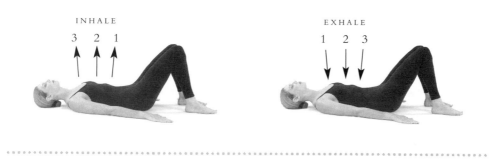

INHALE   EXHALE
3 2 1   1 2 3

Chest-to-Belly Breathing

The ancient technique of Chest-to-Belly Breathing has been popularized in America since the 1970s by the work of T. K. V. Desikachar. Desikachar demonstrated that Chest-to-Belly Breathing is the most effective method for toning muscles along the spine, counteracting the effects of all our sitting and bending forward. It is also very energizing and can be used when you first wake up in the morning or during that afternoon energy lull.

1. As you inhale, expand the chest from the top down, continuing this movement downward into the belly, then pause.
2. As you exhale, slowly draw the belly in, focusing slightly below the navel. Your rib cage will naturally lower. Pause.
3. Repeat 20 to 30 times if you're doing the breathing exercise without movement or as directed in your Yoga therapy routine.

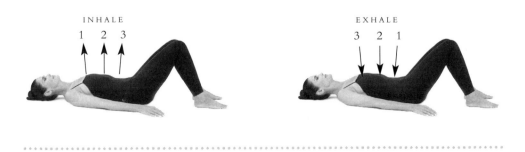

INHALE

1 2 3

EXHALE

3 2 1

Using Sound

The use of sound is a special form of Yoga called Mantra Yoga. You produce sound when air leaving your lungs passes over your vocal cords causing them to vibrate. In Yoga tradition, this vibration creates a healing environment for the body and the mind.

The simple sounds that are user friendly in all languages and dialects are *ah, ma,* and *sa.* They are easy to use and calming to the body and mind. When spoken during an exhale, these sounds substantially lengthen the breath by narrowing the air passages and slowing the release of air from the lungs.

Sound can also help you coordinate your breath and movement. Some people find the Yoga requirement of focusing on the breath to be somewhat abstract. By adding the ability to focus on a sound, they sometimes find the key to success. Tom, a fifty-six-year-old school psychologist, was referred to me by his physician because of numerous stress-related symptoms. He suffered from anxiety, tension headaches, and insomnia. He was an intellectual and an introvert. As he described it, he was "not in his body." He had a difficult time understanding how to link his breath and movement, admitting he was uncoordinated. Feeling that he needed something more concrete to focus on, I suggested that he begin to use sound while doing the Yoga postures. He started with the sound of *ah* for all of the folding movements such as forward bends, side bends, and twists. It was quite a breakthrough. His brain had finally made the connection between his breathing and his action. Soon he was comfortable using any of the three sounds—*ah, ma,* and *sa*—with his Yoga practice. With sound, he could easily coordinate his breath and movement. For the first time in his life, Tom had a physical program that he could do on his own and look forward to. The big payoff was that after three months of regular Yoga practice, all of his stress-related symptoms were gone.

To try using sound, practice any of the four simple breathing techniques outlined earlier, and once you become comfortable, add one of the sounds to your exhale. This means you will be opening your mouth, so you'll be exhaling through your mouth instead of your nose. See if this helps you keep your breath slow and measured and your concentration more intense.

ADVANCED YOGA BREATHING

Now we'll look at five advanced breathing techniques (pranayama in Sanskrit), popularly known as Victorious Breath, Alternate Nostril Breathing, Shining Skull Breath, Cooling Breath, and Crow's Beak. It is important to practice them only after you have become comfortable with the basic Yoga breathing techniques described earlier.

Victorious Breath

Learning the Victorious Breath is traditionally one of the goals of authentic Yogic breathing. It involves producing a sound like an ocean tide or a baby's breath. It is considered a more advanced skill and can be added to any of the Yoga breathing techniques when you are ready.

1. Start seated comfortably or standing with the spine erect.
2. Open your mouth and slowly inhale; as you exhale make a sound at the back of your throat like the ocean's incoming tide or a whispering *haaa*.
3. Now add the sound to your inhale as well. Repeat a few times.
4. Then close your mouth, breathe through the nose on both the inhale and exhale, and make the same sound focusing on the back of your throat and the chest.

Make the breath long and smooth with the normal pauses at the top of the inhale and the bottom of the exhale. It is easier to learn Victorious Breath on the exhale phase. Use this type of breathing to slow yourself down even further and to deepen your concentration.

Alternate Nostril Breathing

Alternate Nostril Breathing (ANB) was developed because Yoga masters knew what researchers have only recently proven in the lab: We don't breath evenly through both nostrils. In a cycle that lasts a few hours, each nostril becomes alternately dominant. ANB helps create balance and harmony in your system by allowing each nostril equal time so that while you are practicing, neither nostril is dominant. This can also help strengthen the breath of a nostril that may be chronically weaker. There are several forms of Alternate Nostril Breathing. The following exercise, called Channel Cleansing, is a safe and popular form of ANB that can easily be practiced by beginners.

1. Sit comfortably in a chair, or on the floor in a simple crossed-legged position. Bring your back up nice and tall.
2. Hold up your right fist with the palm toward you and then extend the right thumb and last two fingers. Your index and middle fingers are folded down.
3. Place your right thumb on the side of your right nostril, and the ring and little fingers on the side of your left nostril.
4. Block off the right nostril and inhale freely into the left. Then block off the left nostril and exhale out of the right. Then reverse it: Inhale into the right nostril while blocking the left, and exhale out of the left while blocking the right.
5. Repeat the cycle 10 to 12 times.

In your first session practicing this technique, start with inhalations and exhalations of five to seven seconds each. Over time as you continue to practice, gradually increase the length of your breath until you reach your comfortable maximum. You can also gradually increase the length of your sessions until you reach five to ten minutes. If a Yoga routine in this book instructs you to do Alternate Nostril Breathing and you have difficulty doing it, you may substitute Belly-to-Chest Breathing or Victorious Breath.

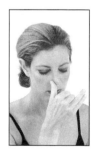

Shining Skull Breath

The Shining Skull Breath exercise has an energizing effect and is great for the physical or mental blahs. In the beginning, this exercise may leave you feeling lightheaded, but it's a great pick-me-up when you need to be alert. During my corporate days, we all had to attend laborious meetings. If I had a hard time staying awake, I would excuse myself for a restroom break, do two or three sets of Shining Skull Breath and come back to the meeting wide awake. The Shining Skull Breath is not recommended just before bedtime, as it may be too stimulating; and it should not be used during pregnancy. The focus is on short rapid inhalations and exhalations using your nose.

1. Sit comfortably in a chair or on the floor in a simple cross-legged position. Bring your back up nice and tall and place your hands on your thighs or in your lap.
2. Take a deep inhale through your nose, then exhale quickly through your nose, strongly contracting your abdominal muscles. Rest your hands on your lower belly to feel the contraction. Let the contraction push the air out of your lungs.
3. Then just as quickly, release the contraction, and watch how the breath is automatically drawn back into your lungs.
4. Repeat this quick contraction–release cycle 15 to 20 times in succession. Each exhalation is about one second.

Go slowly at first; and then after you have practiced for a few days, pick up the pace and add ten to fifteen more cycles. You could also do two sets of cycles, with a ten- to fifteen-second rest between the sets.

Cooling Breath

A great technique for mellowing out during stressful times is the Cooling Breath. It's also effective for quieting hunger or thirst when necessary.

1. Sit in a comfortable position on the floor. Bring your back up nice and tall. Place your hands on your thighs or comfortably on your lap.
2. Curl your tongue vertically and let its tip protrude slightly from your mouth. (The ability to curl your tongue vertically, so that from the front it looks like a U, is genetic. If you can't curl your tongue, try Crow's Beak, described next.)

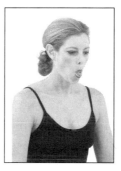

3. As you inhale, slightly tilt your head back while you slowly suck the air in through the funnel formed by your tongue. Then tilt your chin back down as you exhale slowly through your nose.
4. Repeat 10 to 20 times. Gradually increase to 5 to 10 minutes.

Crow's Beak

The Crow's Beak is an alternative if you are unable to curl your tongue for Cooling Breath. This technique has the same benefits as Cooling Breath.

1. Sit in a comfortable position on the floor. Bring your back up nice and tall. Place your hands on your thighs or comfortably in your lap.
2. Pucker your lips as though you were going to suck in air through a straw. As you inhale, slightly tilt your head back while you slowly suck the air in through your puckered lips. Then tilt your chin back down as you exhale slowly through your nose.
3. Repeat 10 to 20 times. Gradually increase to 5 to 10 minutes.

5

Relaxation and Meditation

S tress . . . we've mentioned it several times already, and there's a good
chance it's one of the reasons you're reading this book. Stress is a major factor in our need for the daily calming and healing effects of Yoga. Yoga provides relief from stress through each of its different expressions—postures,
breathing exercises, and especially relaxation and meditation.

What is the difference between relaxation and meditation? The distinction is
subtle but significant. Relaxation is simpler. It usually involves relaxing the physical body, which can take place with an active mind, but ideally quiets the mind as
well. It requires a degree of control over your mind and body, but it is not too difficult. Relaxation is usually something we do to feel better in the moment, like
having a drink or watching TV. Its effects don't extend very far beyond the actual
relaxation time.

Meditation is a deeper, more intense technique in which the meditator seeks not only to reach a deep state of relaxation but also to quiet the mind, and maintain a higher state of being beyond the time of meditation. The process develops the deepest levels of concentration as the practitioner becomes conscious of his or her own awareness and tries to transcend it. Meditation seeks a state of enlightenment, a freedom from the tyranny of our worries. It can be challenging to learn to reach a true state of meditation, but it provides the deepest level of physical and mental relaxation and, consequently, is the most effective for stress reduction.

In this chapter we'll look first at relaxation, then at meditation, giving a few basic techniques for each. Now is the time to think about setting aside ten to fifteen minutes each day to begin practicing these skills. You won't regret it.

RELAXATION

In Sanskrit, the word for relaxation is *shaithilya* (SHY-theel-yah), which translates to "loosening." You can think of relaxation as loosening up your tension, smoothing out all the kinks in your physical, emotional, and mental state. There is much more to relaxation than just "doing nothing." It involves a conscious *effort* to release your body of any *effort*. Sounds paradoxical, and it is; that's why relaxation is a skill to be cultivated.

When you're getting ready to begin relaxation exercises, try to be in a quiet environment where you're unlikely to be disturbed. Wear appropriate clothing to make sure you are comfortable and just the right temperature—you don't want to be too warm or too cold. In addition, don't practice on a full stomach. After a heavy meal, wait two to three hours.

The Quickie

Of all the relaxation techniques, the Quickie is the simplest and the fastest. According to Yoga's esoteric anatomy, the left nostril is part of the "channel of comfort," which is one of the three main energy flows in the human body. It is associated with the energy of the moon. Simply breathing deeply into the left side will often create a calming effect.

1. Sit comfortably in a chair with your back straight.
2. Bring your right elbow close to your rib cage and block the right side of your nostril with your right thumb, or use the hand position recommended for Alternate Nostril Breathing (page 45).
3. Breathe slowly and deeply through the left nostril only, for 3 to 5 minutes. Make your breath a little longer than normal, and be sure to pause after the inhale and the exhale.
4. When you're finished, bring the right hand down, let your breath come back to normal, and get up slowly.

Stress Buster

The Stress Buster relaxation technique is especially good for that stressful time in the afternoon at the office, or just before bed to help you go to sleep. If you are at the office, close the door to ensure privacy. Wherever you are, turn off the phone and do what you can to prevent disturbances. You will need a chair, a small towel or eye bag to cover your eyes, and one or two blankets.

1. Lie on your back on the floor with your feet up on the seat of a chair. Make sure that your legs are about hip-width apart and supported by the seat of the chair all the way to the back of your knees.
2. If your head tilts back, place a blanket under your head. Cover your eyes with a towel or eye bag. Unless the room is warm, cover your body with a blanket from neck to toes.
3. Bring your focus to your belly. Breathing through the nose as you inhale, expand the belly slowly in all directions (top, bottom, sides). Once you are comfortable with Belly Breathing (page 41), begin to gradually increase the length of your exhalation until you reach your comfortable maximum. (Inhale freely, exhale forever.)
4. Repeat for 5 to 10 minutes. When you are finished, let your breath come back to normal, and rest for at least 1 minute before getting up.

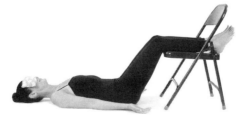

Healing Triangles

Relaxation techniques such as this one involve directing your awareness to specific parts of your body, which means you have to control your thoughts. In this way, some relaxation exercises come close to resembling meditation.

1. Sit in a chair comfortably with your back straight.
2. Take a few deep breaths and then settle in to your normal breathing through your nose.
3. Bring your focus mentally to the middle of your forehead and begin to draw a mental triangle between your forehead and the palms of both hands. See the triangle in your mind and if any part is difficult to connect (usually the bottom), spend some time there and then try to reconnect the entire triangle. Stay for 15 breaths. Then release the triangle and breathe normally.
4. When you are comfortable with one triangle, see if you can hold the triangle in your mind and then at the same time mentally connect a second triangle using your navel and the big toes of both feet.
5. Try to hold both of the triangles for 3 to 5 minutes. Release the first triangle, then the second and breathe normally.
6. As a long-range goal, once you can hold two triangles in your mind try for a third. Mentally connect with a point of light just above your head (sometimes called an infinity point). See the light separating and going down the outside of your body below your feet. The third triangle surrounds the other two. The third triangle may be very large, or close to your body. When you reach the point of holding three triangles, try to continue for 5 to 20 minutes.

This exercise is not easy and takes time to learn. The more you practice, the easier it will be, as in the process of building up a muscle. You may notice colors forming in the triangles, or sensations inside of the triangles—mental, emotional, or physical. Just observe. When you are ready to end the exercise, release the triangles in the order you created them. Then let the breath come back to normal and relax for a while.

Yoga Nidra

Yoga Nidra literally means "Yoga sleep." Although there are many variations of Yoga Nidra, the most popular is used to facilitate a deep state of relaxation, which is very conducive to healing. When they are not otherwise engaged, the systems of the body are free to replenish and heal. Think of Yoga Nidra as a natural tranquilizer, leading to mental, physical, and emotional harmony. Although Yoga Nidra can be practiced anytime and anywhere, the best times are early morning and just before sleep.

Yoga Nidra traditionally incorporates a positive affirmation, a visualization, and a systematic rotation of consciousness to specific parts of the body. Before practicing the routine, consider having someone read the copy to you while you do the relaxation, or record yourself reading the instructions. (It will be difficult to relax fully if you are trying to read at the same time.) Later you will be able to do the routine from memory. An excellent source on Yoga Nidra is available by Richard Miller (see Resource Guide).

1. *Preparation:* Lie on your back comfortably in the Corpse pose—bring your arms across your chest and hug yourself. Now let your elbows come down to the floor, then let the forearms and the back of your hands flop down to a comfortable place with palms up. Slowly turn your head from side to side and then back to the middle.
2. Close your eyes. Take a few deep breaths through the nose and then continue normal breathing through the nose.
3. *First resolve:* Either mentally or verbally make a sincere statement about improving your health or your life, while continuing to breathe normally. Pause before moving on to the next mental step. (Each pause in this exercise should last about 10 seconds.)
4. *Visualization:* As you inhale, visualize the healing rays of the sun warming and healing your entire body or, specifically, an injured or affected area. As you exhale, visualize darkness, impurities, and ill-health leaving the body.
5. Repeat for 15 to 30 breaths. Then slowly bring your focus back to the moment.

6. *Rotation of consciousness:* Bring your attention to the bottom of your feet and begin to relax your toes one at a time, beginning with the big toes on both feet, then the next toe, the next, the next, and the little toe. Pause. Release your ankles and then your knees. Mentally go inside of your knees and look around. Visualize tendons and ligaments. Imagine the kneecaps from underneath. Breathe into your knees and mentally instruct your knees to relax. Pause. Move your focus to your thighs and begin to visualize breathing into your thighs. Deeper, deeper until you reach the hamstrings underneath. Visualize the hamstrings releasing, relaxing, letting go. Pause. Now release the hips into the floor. Just let go. Pause. Bring your focus to your lower back. Think about the connection with your lower back, the floor, and the earth. Pause. Bring that same connection to the middle and upper back.

7. Breathe into any tight spots (or visualize your prana flowing to these places). If you feel any tension, let it go. Pause. Surrender your shoulders down through the arms, down through the hands, and out through your fingertips. Pause. Release the back of your head and all of the tight spots behind the ears. Pause. Move your attention to your face, starting with the tight spot between the eyes. Now relax the muscles around your eyes, the nose, and the mouth. Release the mouth, the tongue, the spot below the tongue, just let it go. Pause.

8. (Option) You can repeat the rotation sequence (Steps 6 and 7) 1 to 3 more times, depending on the time you have available and how deeply you want to relax.

9. *Remember the feeling:* Take a few moments to think about how you're feeling right now, in your body and in your mind. Try to hold this feeling so that you will remember it later. Wiggle your toes and fingers, open the eyes a little, then a little more. Bring your arms overhead and stretch out. Roll to one side and stay there for a while. When you come up, let your head be the last thing to rise up. Use your hands, arms, and forearms to push up into a sitting position, and then relax until you are ready for your next activity.

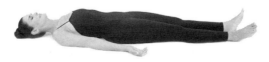

MEDITATION

If someone offered you a quick do-it-yourself drug-free way to lower stress and reduce pain, would you be interested? With stress and pain under control, many people report improved memory, concentration, creativity, and productivity. These may sound like the some of the same benefits of Yoga you've already read about in this book. But meditation offers these advantages without requiring exercise. Great results can be achieved in only ten to twenty minutes of meditation a day or several sessions a week. Meditation does not require any special props, equipment, or clothing, plus—like Yoga breathing and relaxation—once the skill is acquired, you can take it with you anywhere.

Is meditation a required part of your Yoga practice? Not necessarily, but if you're reading this book, you probably have health concerns; and like the Yoga breathing discussed in Chapter 4 and the relaxation exercises presented in this chapter, meditation is just one more powerful tool for restoring your body to optimum health. Meditating brings you into a deep state of calm, soothing the central nervous system and releasing the mind from worries. This encourages your systems to work at their full capacities to help your body heal itself.

By now you're catching on to the possible benefits of meditation, but now we must direct your attention to the fine print: There's nothing easy about it. If you aren't accustomed to sitting quietly and doing absolutely nothing except being with yourself, even a short meditation can seem as tough as a climb up Mount Everest. You will probably encounter the gremlins, the ones that make your nose itch, your back ache, your brain race, and your foot fall asleep—all the little things that will drive you to distraction. Like any worthy endeavor, meditation requires commitment, patience, and a healthy measure of perseverance.

After ten years of learning and teaching Yoga, I asked a great meditation teacher to help me develop a deeper meditation practice. I decided to focus on meditating during one of my annual trips to the garden island of Kauai. My teacher's most important bit of advice was simple: No matter how distracted the mind is, be patient and sit three times a day, beginning with five minutes and working toward a goal of thirty minutes at a time.

On the first morning, I plunged in, telling myself, "I am going to sit here for half an hour if it kills me." Well, it almost did! I couldn't believe how difficult it was to sit quietly for even five minutes. My mind was going everywhere, a common circumstance that I later learned is called "monkey mind." But I remembered my teacher's advice. As challenging as it was, I sat there and focused on my breathing.

By the third day, I was learning to be more patient. I set smaller goals, and soon I was able to sit with a relatively quiet mind for five whole minutes. As I increased my goal in tiny increments, I found I was able to sit quietly for longer each session. When we approach our goals this way, things that might have seemed unthinkable become real possibilities.

A meditative state is often compared to a tranquil body of water, such as a placid lake or pond. What is less often said, however, is that once tranquility is achieved, it doesn't necessarily guarantee that only calm or positive feelings come to the surface. To extend the lake analogy, there may very well be debris at the bottom that floats up in the form of negative thoughts or feelings, perhaps anger, resentment, or discontent. When you first try meditation, you might also feel bored, sleepy, or a general discomfort. This is a common response; try to acknowledge those thoughts and feelings without judging them. It's all part of the journey leading us to the ultimate goal of meditation: to quiet our minds enough to hear our inner voice, seek true wisdom, and experience our deepest intuition. Along the way to these somewhat lofty ideals, remember that simple meditation and relaxation techniques are among the best ways to manage stress.

Meditation Techniques

Meditation can take years to master, but you don't have to be an expert to reap rewards. You will see benefits even if you never progress past these three basic meditation techniques: Focused, Open-Ended, and Mantra.

. . . .

Focused Meditation

Focused Meditation is a technique in which you direct your awareness onto something. It could be an object like a picture or statue of a deity; a universal principle such as compassion or forgiveness; or a symbol such as *om*, the famous Hindu mantra.

You can try Focused Meditation right now. Just be aware that this elementary exercise isn't as easy as it seems, so be patient and compassionate with yourself.

One of the favorite objects of meditation is your own breath. It's certainly convenient, and the Yogis maintain it's a direct channel to your authentic self.

1. Sit comfortably, close your eyes, and begin to focus on your inhalation and your exhalation

2. As you inhale through your nose, count to yourself, "One." Exhale. Then, on the next inhale, count, "Two," And so on. After each inhalation, try to hold your breath for one short beat before the exhalation. That short, quiet pause may serve as a doorway into meditation because at that point you are close to stillness.

How high can you count before you lose track of the count completely? Be honest with yourself. Don't be shocked if you forget the count fairly quickly. Just go back to square one and start again. Keep trying until you can count straight through to ten, and if you get to ten, go back and count to ten again. Notice what happens to your breath as you focus on it for increasingly longer counts, and what effect this has on your awareness. Strengthening your ability to focus is just like strengthening a muscle. The more you exercise your awareness, the stronger it gets.

. . . .

Open-Ended Meditation

Open-Ended Meditation is a technique in which there's no particular object of meditation. The meditator just opens up to his or her own inner experience and simply observes whatever arises, without identifying with or judging that experience.

Again, it's not hard to begin this kind of meditation, though at first it is difficult to stay with it for more than a minute or so.

1. Sit comfortably and close your eyes. Bring your awareness to your thoughts, feelings, fantasies, desires, memories—whatever comes up for you. Don't get attached to what comes up, and don't try to direct it, just be an observer and witness to it all.

2. As you progress and are able to hang on to this open-ended awareness for longer periods of time, notice what happens to the usual flood of contents that continually swirls around inside your head. Practice this until you feel comfortable maintaining it for at least 5 minutes.

Mantra Meditation

In Sanskrit, the *man* in mantra means "to think," and the *tra* suggests "instrumentality." *Mantra* literally means an "instrument of thought." The whole idea with mantra meditation is to repeat a word, phrase, or sound to transcend the constant distractions of the mind. The continuous repetition of a mantra is called japa. The concept of mantra can be found in many spiritual traditions, including Christianity, Hinduism, Buddhism, and Judaism. Millions of Americans were introduced to Mantra Yoga in the 1960s through the Transcendental Meditation (TM) movement founded by Maharishi Mahesh Yogi of India.

1. To begin, choose a word, phrase, or a short sentence from a prayer or poem that inspires you. For example, you could choose the sentence, "Thou art with me," from Psalm 23. Limit your mantra to three or four words at the most.
2. Sit quietly in a chair with your back up straight. Close your eyes or half close them, gazing downward. Take a few deep breaths through the nose.
3. When you're ready, say the mantra you have chosen during your exhale. Continue to inhale through your nose, and repeat your mantra out loud on each exhalation, for 5 to 10 minutes.

You will have more success with your concentration if you can hear yourself verbalizing your mantra. After you've been practicing for some time, you may want to begin reciting the mantra very softly or even silently, as this is said to be the most powerful form of mantra meditation. Once you feel comfortable with the silent recitation, begin repeating the mantra mentally with your thoughts during both the inhale and the exhale. You can use this form of meditation for up to thirty minutes.

6

Core Yoga Routines That

Really Heal

Are you ready to do some Yoga? Now that you've become familiar with Yoga breathing, relaxation, and meditation, it's time to learn some basic postures and do your first Yoga routine.

There is no single posture or Yoga routine that is right for everyone. Yoga therapy is based on adapting a program to fit the needs of the individual. However, there are basic principles and safe routines commonly used for general conditioning and for treatment of selected health conditions. The two Yoga routines in this chapter are designed to help your body heal itself. Core Routine I is designed to help beginners bring the body into balance with strength and flexibility, and Core Routine II is a bit more advanced and helps build stamina. They are a gentle introduction to Yoga and a great place for you to start if you're ready for general conditioning. If Core Routine I seems a bit difficult, start with the Lower Back Routine (page 114), which is even more gentle and helps balance your body. If you have a specific ailment that is addressed in Part III, please do the routine recommended in that chapter.

I hope that you've read Chapters 1 through 5 already, but it is particularly important that you read Chapter 3 on getting started, and Chapter 4 on Yoga Breathing before trying any of these routines.

Photographs of Yoga postures are shown in the modified form with forgiving limbs—feet placed at hip width, legs and arms slightly bent. This is inspired by the Viniyoga tradition, which seeks to adapt the Yoga postures to fit the needs of the person, and ensures that you will be safe and kind to your body while learning Yoga techniques. As mentioned in Chapter 3, these postures may look different from the classic Yoga poses you have seen, which in many cases are too extreme for the average Yoga practitioner.

CORE ROUTINE I

You should use Focused Breathing (page 39) for the whole routine. Move slowly, and remember the brief pauses after the inhale and the exhale.

Caution: If any of the postures cause pain or do not feel right, simply leave them out and check with your health-care professional before continuing.

....

Mountain Posture

The Mountain Posture is the cornerstone for all standing postures, and you will be using it throughout this routine. It improves posture and spinal alignment, creating stability in your stance and facilitating breathing.

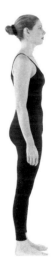

1. Stand with your feet at hip width. Keep your spine tall but relaxed. Let your arms hang at your sides, palms turned inward toward your legs.
2. Align the middle of your ear, your shoulder, and the sides of your hip, knee, and ankle along an imaginary vertical line.
3. Look straight ahead.
4. Remain in this posture for 8 to 10 breaths.

Standing Forward Bend

This posture stretches the entire backside of your body, including your neck, shoulders, back, and hamstrings. It promotes circulation to your upper trunk and head, and adds flexibility to your spine.

Caution: If you have been diagnosed with a spinal problem (such as a herniated disk), acute hypertension, or glaucoma, be careful of all standing forward bends. Avoid this posture if it causes you any pain.

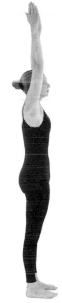

1. Begin in the Mountain Posture. As you inhale, raise your arms from the front, up and overhead.
2. As you exhale, bend forward from your hips, bringing your arms, hands, torso, and head forward and down toward the floor. When you feel a pull in the back of your legs, soften your knees and hang your arms.
3. As you inhale, choose one of three ways to come up, listed here in order of increasing difficulty.
   a. Roll up like a rag doll, stacking the vertebrae one at a time, and then raise your arms forward and up as in Step 1.
   b. Sweep your arms up from the sides like wings until your arms are overhead and your head and torso are straight up as in Step 1.
   c. Bring your arms and hands forward and up alongside your ears and then bring your arms, head, and torso up as in Step 1.
4. Repeat 3 times, and then hold Step 2 for 6 to 8 breaths. Come up a final time.

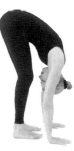

Warrior I

This lunge-like posture strengthens your legs, back, shoulders, and arms. It helps improve stamina and balance and increases flexibility in your hips.

1. Start in the Mountain Posture. Take a big step forward with your right foot, approximately 3 feet for taller people, less if you are shorter. Your right knee should be directly over your ankle, and your thigh should be parallel to the floor. Place your hands on your hips and square your hips forward. Keep both legs straight and hang your arms at your sides in the ready position.
2. As you inhale, raise your arms forward and up overhead, and at the same time bend your right knee to a right angle. You should feel like you're in a classic runner's stretch, with a light pull in your left calf.
3. As you exhale, straighten your right leg and bring your arms back to the ready position as in Step 1.
4. Repeat 3 times, then hold Step 2 for 6 to 8 breaths. Straighten up.
5. Repeat on the left side

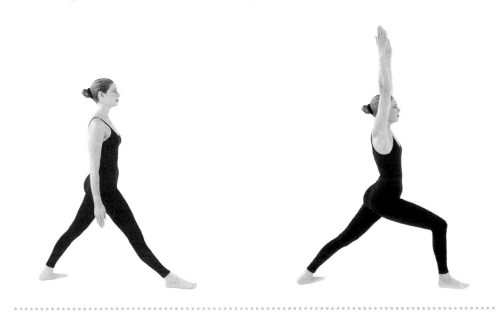

Standing Asymmetrical Forward Bend

This posture stretches each side of your hips, hamstrings, and back.

1. Start in the Mountain Posture. Take a big step forward with your right foot, approximately 3 feet for taller people, less if you are shorter. Place your hands on your hips and rotate your torso toward the right, squaring your hips forward. Bend your right knee but keep your torso straight up. Check your stance. Make sure your knee is above your ankle so that your shin is perpendicular to the floor, your thigh parallel, and your knee at a right angle. Finally, straighten both legs, and hang your arms at your sides in the ready position.

2. As you inhale, raise your arms, stretching them forward and up alongside your ears.

3. As you exhale, bend from your hips, forward and down, over your front leg. Soften your front leg to fit your needs. If your head is not close to your right leg, bend your right knee more. If you have the flexibility, straighten your right leg, pull your right hip back and your left hip forward.

4. On the inhalation, choose one of three ways to come up:
   a. Roll up like a rag doll, stacking your vertebrae one at a time, and then raise your arms forward and up as in Step 2.
   b. Sweep your arms up from the sides like wings until your arms are overhead and your head and torso are straight up as in Step 2.
   c. Bring your arms and hands forward and up alongside of your ears and then bring your arms, head, and torso up as in Step 2.

5. Repeat Steps 3 and 4, three times. The last time, stay in the folded position for 6 to 8 breaths, then roll up as described in Step 4a.

6. Return to the Mountain Posture, and repeat on the left side.

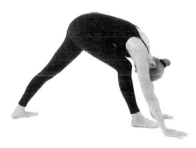

Revolved Triangle

This gentle twisting posture stimulates circulation to your spine, opens your hips, and stretches your hamstrings and calves. It also strengthens your neck, shoulders, and arms.

1. Start in the Mountain Posture. Exhaling, step out to the right in a wide stance, approximately 3 feet for taller people, less if you are shorter, still facing forward.
2. As you inhale, raise your arms out to the sides, parallel to the floor forming a T.
3. Exhaling, bend forward from your hips; then, in a twisting motion, place your right palm or fingers on the floor near the inside of your left foot. Continue exhaling. Raise your left arm into a vertical position and look up at your left hand. To make the posture easier, soften your left knee and arms, or move your right hand back to the right, below the midline of your torso. To make the posture more challenging, straighten your leg and place your right hand just outside of your left foot. Return to the upright position.
4. Repeat 3 times, and then hold Step 3 for 6 to 8 breaths.
5. Repeat the same sequence on the other side. When finished, return to the Mountain Posture.

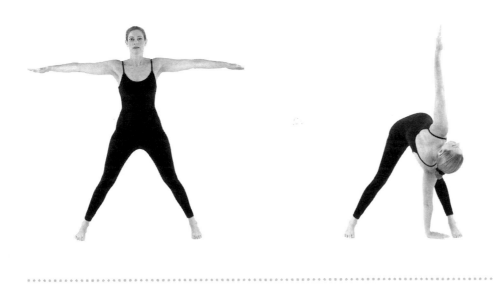

Standing Spread-Leg Forward Bend

This forward bend stimulates circulation to your upper torso and head. It opens your hips and stretches the backs and insides of your legs, including your hamstrings and adductors.

1. Start in the Mountain Posture. Step out to the right with your right foot in a wide stance, approximately 3 feet for taller people, less if you are shorter. As you inhale, raise your arms out from the sides forming a T with your torso.

2. As you exhale, bend forward from the hips and hang down, holding each of your bent elbows with the opposite side hand. Soften your knees to where you are comfortable.

3. Stay in the folded position for 6 to 8 breaths. Roll your body up and return to the Mountain Posture.

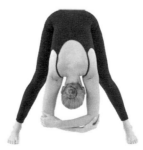

The Willow

This side-bending posture stretches the lateral muscles of your trunk and laterally flexes your spine.

1. Start in the Mountain Posture. As you inhale, rotate your palms out to the sides and bring your arms up and overhead. Touch your palms together with your arms alongside your ears. Keep your shoulders dropped. You should feel your shoulder blades pressing in toward each other.
2. As you inhale, stretch your spine and arms upward.
3. As you exhale, soften your knees and bend your upper torso, arms, and head to the right. Soften your knees more to make the posture easier or straighten your knees to make it more challenging.
4. As you inhale, return to the vertical position. As you exhale again, repeat to the left side.
5. Alternate each side 3 times, then stay on each side for 6 to 8 breaths. Return to the vertical position.

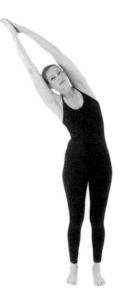

Standing Forward Bend

Repeating the posture deepens the stretch on the entire backside of your body, including your neck, shoulders, back, and hamstrings.

Caution: If you have been diagnosed with a spinal problem (such as a herniated disk), acute hypertension, or glaucoma be careful of all standing forward bends. Avoid this posture if it causes you any pain.

1. Begin in the Mountain Posture. As you inhale, raise your arms from the front, up and overhead.
2. As you exhale, bend forward from your hips, bringing your arms, hands, torso, and head forward and down toward the floor. When you feel a pull in the back of your legs, soften your knees and hang your arms.
3. As you inhale, choose one of three ways to come up:
   a. Roll up like a rag doll, stacking the vertebrae one at a time, and then raise your arms forward and up as in Step 1.
   b. Sweep your arms up from the sides like wings until your arms are overhead and your head and torso are straight up as in Step 1.
   c. Bring your arms and hands forward and up alongside your ears and then bring your arms, head, and torso up as in Step 1.
4. Repeat 3 times, and then hold Step 2 for 6 to 8 breaths. Come up a final time.

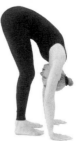

The Tree

This posture improves focus, concentration, balance, and stability. It increases the flexibility of your hips and groin, and strengthens your legs.

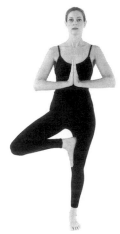

1. Stand in the Mountain Posture. As you exhale, place the sole of your left foot on the inside of your right leg above your knee, toes pointing toward the ground.
2. As you inhale, bring your arms out from your sides to form a T, and then, as you exhale, bring your hands together in prayer position with your thumbs touching your breastbone and fingers toward the ceiling. As a variation, bring your arms overhead and join your palms together. Look at a spot on the floor 6 to 8 feet in front of you.
3. Stay for 6 to 8 breaths and then repeat on the other side.

The Corpse

This is the classic posture for relaxation of your body and mind. It can also be used for deep relaxation and treatment for hypertension.

1. Lie flat on your back with your arms relaxed near your sides and palms turned up. Close your eyes and relax. If your head tilts back or your neck is uncomfortable, place a small pillow or blanket under your head and neck. If your lower back is uncomfortable, place a pillow or rolled blanket under your knees.
2. Stay in the position for 8 to 10 breaths.

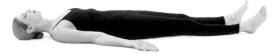

Note: This is the halfway point of the routine.
If you have only fifteen minutes, you can stop here.

Abdominal Flow

This is a good strengthener for your lower abs and lower back.

1. Lie on your back with your knees bent, feet flat on the floor at hip width. Interlace your fingers behind your head with your elbows wide and open.
2. As you inhale, raise your hips off the floor as high as you feel comfortable, stretching your back muscles.
3. As you exhale, bring your hips down and then fold your body by bringing your chest, head, and knees toward each other, curling your chin into your chest. Keep your eyes focused on your knees. Try to keep your elbows wide.
4. Repeat Steps 1 to 3 slowly, 6 to 8 times.

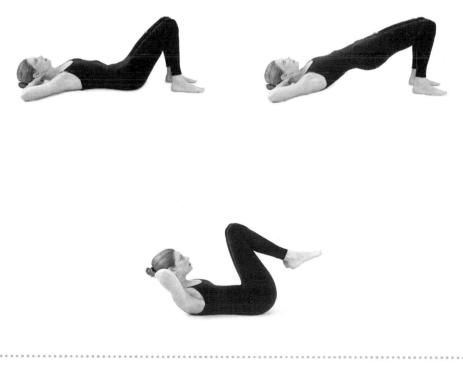

Cobra (Kite Variation)

The Cobra increases the flexibility and strength of your arms, chest, shoulders, and back. It also opens your chest and increases lung capacity.

1. Lie on your belly, with your forehead on the floor, legs slightly apart with the tops of your feet on the floor. Relax your arms at your sides, palms up. If you have lower back problems, separate your legs wider than your hips, and turn your heels out and toes in.
2. Inhaling, raise your chest, engaging your back muscles. Sweep your arms from the sides like wings until you reach a T position in line with your shoulders.
3. Exhaling, lower your torso, head, and arms back to the floor as in Step 1.
4. Repeat 6 to 8 times.

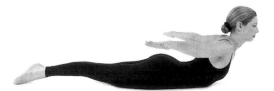

Child's Posture

This is a gentle stretch for your lower back, helping it relax and loosen up any tension. It is often used as a compensation posture after back bends or back stretches, which is how we're using it here.

1. Start on your hands and knees with the heels of your hands directly below your shoulders and your knees at hip width. Look down slightly.
2. As you exhale, sit back on your heels. Relax in the posture, and try to rest your torso on your thighs and your forehead on the floor. Do not force yourself beyond your comfort zone.
3. Rest your arms at your sides, palms up. Close your eyes. Breathe easily.
4. Stay for 6 to 8 breaths.

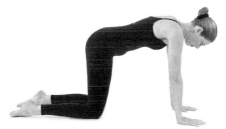

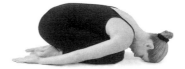

Hamstring Stretch

This stretch feels great on your hamstrings and prepares your body for numerous sitting, kneeling, and standing postures.

1. Lie on your back with your knees bent, feet on the floor at hip width. Slide your right leg all the way down, and relax your arms at your sides, palms down.
2. As you exhale, bring your right leg up to a comfortable height. (Draw your belly in as you are exhaling to make more room for your right leg to come up.)
3. As you inhale, bring your leg back down.
4. Repeat 3 times. On the last leg raise, clasp the back of your right thigh just below your knee with both hands interlaced, hold for 6 to 8 breaths. Lower your leg.
5. Repeat on the left side.

Do not force it. Your leg does not need to be fully extended in the beginning. Keep your head and the top of your hips on the floor. Place a pillow or blanket under your head if it tilts back.

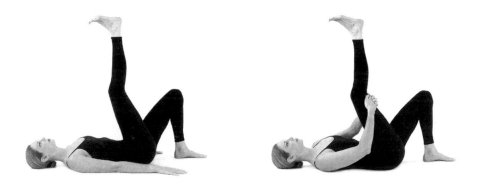

Seated Forward Bend

Caution: If you have a problem with an intervertebral disk, be especially careful of all straight-leg, seated forward bends. Try modifying by bending your knees and keeping your back extended and chest lifted. Avoid rounding your back. If it hurts, do not do this posture.

1. Sit on the floor, with your legs extended in front of you at hip width. Place your hands, palms down, on the floor near your thighs. Lift your chest and bring your back up nice and tall, as if a string attached to the top of your head were lifting you to the sky.
2. As you inhale, raise your arms from the front, up and overhead until they are parallel with your ears. Keep your arms and legs soft and slightly bent.
3. As you exhale, bend forward from your hips. Extend your hands, chest, and head toward your legs. Place your hands on your legs, feet, or the floor. If your head is not close to your knees, soften your knees until you feel your back stretching. To make the posture more challenging, bring your chest forward toward your feet, extending your back and straightening your legs more. As you inhale, raise your arms, head, and torso until you are in the upright position as in Step 2.
4. Repeat 3 times, then stay folded (as in Step 3) for 6 to 8 breaths.

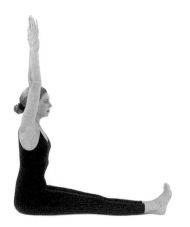
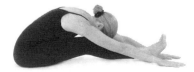

Sage Twist

This simple twisting motion stretches and strengthens your abs and promotes healthy digestion.

1. Sit flat on the floor, with your legs extended in front of you at hip width. Bend your right knee and place the right foot on the floor with the heel near your groin, parallel to and 4 to 6 inches from your left thigh.
2. Place your right palm on the floor behind you, near your tailbone. Turn your fingers away from your hips. Bend your left arm and place your left elbow outside of your right knee with your fingers pointing up.
3. As you inhale, lift your chest and head, bringing your back up nice and tall. As you exhale, rotate your shoulders and upper back to the right.
4. Repeat for 3 breaths, gradually increasing the twist. Then stay in your comfortable maximum twist for 6 to 8 breaths.
5. Return to the upright position with your legs extended in front of you, then repeat on the left side.

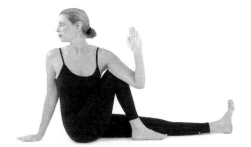

Knees to Chest

This posture relieves stiffness, misalignment, and discomfort in your lower back. It releases abdominal gas and relieves menstrual cramps. We are using it to compensate for the twisting of your back in the previous posture. (Note that the Knees to Chest is different from the Knee to Chest, which appears elsewhere in the book.)

1. Lie on your back with your knees bent, feet on the floor at hip width. Bring your bent knees toward your chest and hold on to the top of your shins, just below your knees, one hand on each knee. If you are having knee problems, hold the backs of your thighs, under your knees.
2. As you exhale, draw your knees toward your chest. As you inhale, move your knees a few inches away from your chest, rolling your hips to the floor.
3. Repeat 3 times, and then stay in the most folded position for 6 to 8 breaths.
4. Return your feet to the floor, then straighten your legs and relax in the Corpse posture.

Relaxation Technique

Remain in the Corpse Posture. Choose one of the relaxation techniques from Chapter 5 and do it for at least 3 to 5 minutes.

CORE ROUTINE II

Use Chest-to-Belly Breathing (page 42) or Belly-to-Chest Breathing (page 41) for the whole routine. Move slowly and remember the brief pauses after the inhale and the exhale.

Caution: If any of the postures cause pain or do not feel right, simply leave them out. Check with your health-care professional before continuing.

....

Mountain Posture

The Mountain Posture is the cornerstone for all standing postures, and you will be using it throughout this routine. It improves posture and spinal alignment, creating stability in your stance and facilitating breathing.

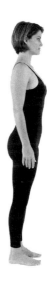

1. Stand with your feet at hip width. Keep your spine tall but relaxed. Let your arms hang at your sides, palms turned inward toward your legs.
2. Align the middle of your ear, your shoulder, and the sides of your hip, knee, and ankle along an imaginary vertical line.
3. Look straight ahead.
4. Remain in this posture for 8 to 10 breaths.

Sun Salutation

The Sun Salutation is a sequence of postures that stretches and supports your spine and improves posture and coordination.

1. Start at the front of your mat or space in the Mountain Posture. Place your palms together in the prayer position with the back of your thumbs touching your sternum in the middle of your chest with your fingers pointing up.

2. As you inhale, extend your hands and arms forward, then up overhead (upward salute). Look at the ceiling and arch your back gently.

3. As you exhale, bend forward from your hips, soften your knees (forgiving limbs), and place your fingers or hands on the floor. Bring your head as close as possible to your legs.

4. As you inhale, step your right foot back into a lunge and bend your left knee. Your left knee should be directly over your ankle (at a right angle) and your thigh should be parallel to the floor. Gaze straight ahead.

5. As you exhale, bring your left foot back even with the right and hold a push-up position. If your arms are not strong enough, you can rest briefly on your hands and knees.

6. Inhale, and then as you exhale, bring your knees, chest, and chin to the floor, leaving your buttocks raised.

7. Inhaling, slide your chest forward along the floor, and then arch back into the Cobra posture. Keep your shoulders dropped and elbows in.

8. Exhaling, turn your toes under, lift your hips up, extend your legs as much as possible, and bring your chest down. Keep both palms on the floor. Your head should be in alignment with your arms. Look behind you at your feet.

9. As you inhale, bring your right foot forward between your hands and gaze straight ahead. Your shin should be at a right angle to the floor.

10. As you exhale, bring your left foot forward, even with your right. Soften your knees and fold into a standing forward bend, as in Step 3.

11. As you inhale, raise your arms in either of the following positions. Then arch back and look up, as in Step 2.
    a. Forward and up overhead from the front.
    b. Out and up from the sides like wings.
12. As you exhale, bring your hands back to the prayer position, as in Step 1.
13. Repeat the entire sequence for 3 to 10 rounds. First lead with your right foot, and then with your left foot, alternating for an equal number of times (each side counts as half a round).

To make the sequence more challenging, execute three to six full rounds and then during the normal cycle, hold for six to eight extra breaths in Steps 2, 3, 4, 5, 7, 8, and 9. Move slowly, pausing after the inhalation and the exhalation.

If you have minor back problems that are aggravated by lifting up from the forward bend in Step 11, try rolling your torso up. Keep your chin on your chest as you roll up, stacking your vertebrae one at a time, while your arms hang at your sides. Once you are fully upright, bring your arms up and overhead from the front or the sides, arch back just a little, and look up. (If your back isn't bothering you, don't use this variation, since it doesn't work your back as thoroughly.)

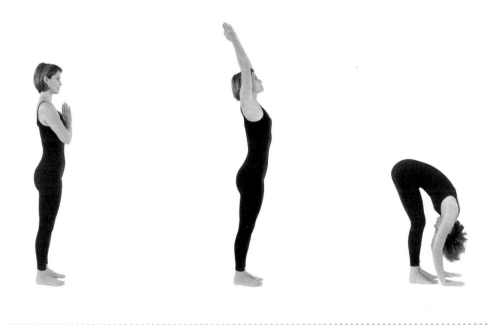

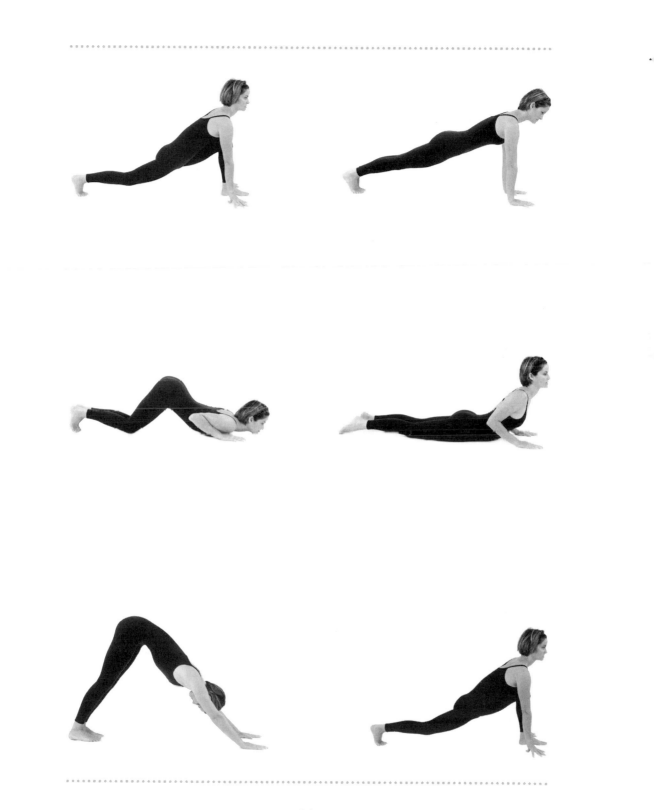

Revolved Triangle

The Revolved Triangle is great for strengthening your neck and stretching out your back and hamstrings.

1. Start in the Mountain Posture. Exhaling, step out to the right in a wide stance, approximately 3 feet for taller people, less if you are shorter.
2. As you inhale, raise your arms out to the sides, parallel to the floor, forming a T.
3. Exhaling, bend forward from your hips and then in a twisting motion, place your right palm or fingers on the floor near the inside of your left foot.
4. Continuing to exhale, raise your left arm into a vertical position and look up at your left hand.

To make the posture easier, soften your knees and arms or bend your left knee and move your right hand closer to the middle of your torso on the floor. To make the posture more challenging, straighten your legs and place your right hand just outside of your left foot.

5. Repeat 3 times. Then stay in Step 4 for 6 to 8 breaths.
6. Repeat the same sequence on the left side. When finished, return to the Mountain Posture.

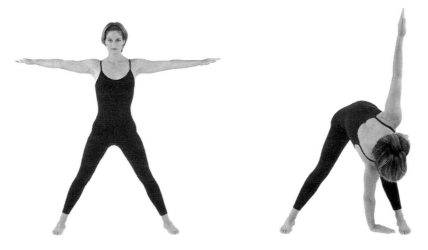

Standing Spread-Leg Forward Bend II

This forward bend stretches the back of your body, especially your spine and legs. It is also good for stretching your neck muscles.

1. Start in the Mountain Posture. Exhaling, step out to the right with your right foot in a wide stance, 3 to 4 feet, depending on your size. Clasp your hands behind your back and interlace your fingers with your palms together.
2. As you inhale, lift your chest and pull your shoulders and arms back.
3. As you exhale, bend forward from your hips and bring your arms over your head as far as they want to go. Be careful not to force this posture.
4. Roll up, leading with your chest. Repeat 3 times. Then hold the forward position for 6 to 8 breaths, keeping your hands together behind your back.

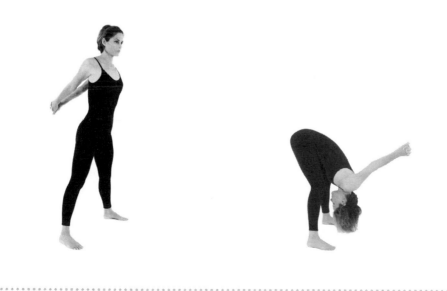

Warrior III

This posture strengthens your legs, back, shoulders, and arms, building stamina. It opens your hips and chest, and improves balance. It is called the Warrior in reference to its Sanskrit namesake, a famous warrior.

1. Start in the Mountain Posture. As you inhale, raise your arms from the front, up and overhead alongside your ears.
2. As you exhale, begin to slide the left foot back, bringing your heel off the floor. Bend forward from your hips with your arms extended forward, and lift your back foot off the floor until your torso, arms, and back leg are parallel with the floor. Your arms and ears should stay in alignment, and you should feel your weight balancing on your front foot. Pick a spot on the floor to focus on 6 to 8 feet in front of you.
3. Hold this position for 6 to 8 breaths; then return to upright in the Mountain Posture.
4. Repeat, pushing the other leg back.

In the beginning, stop bending forward at any point you are unable to keep your balance. Gradually, move closer and closer to the parallel position.

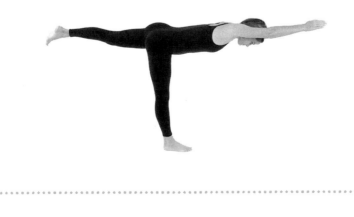

The Corpse

We use this posture to relax in the middle of a routine and/or at the end of one.

1. Lie flat on your back with your arms relaxed near your sides and palms turned up. Close your eyes and relax. If your head tilts back or your neck is uncomfortable, place a small pillow or blanket under your head and neck. If your lower back is uncomfortable, bend your knees and place your feet on the floor at hip width. You could also try putting a rolled blanket or bolster under your knees.
2. Hold this position for 8 to 10 breaths.

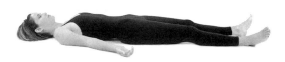

This is the halfway point of the routine.
If you have only fifteen minutes, you can stop here.

The Boat

This posture is excellent for improving balance and working your abs.

1. Sit with your legs fully extended in front of you. Place your hands on the floor behind you at a comfortable distance, with your fingers pointing toward your hips and with your arms straight. Lean your torso slightly back and lift your chest but keep your shoulders down.

2. As you exhale, raise your right leg as high as comfortable, without losing the lift in your chest. Then bring both arms and hands forward until they are stretched out in front of you, parallel to each other and the floor.

3. When you're ready, bring your left leg up beside the right, or you can lower the right before lifting the left. To make the posture more challenging, lift your legs (or leg) to a level slightly above your head. Stay for 6 to 8 breaths, either with both legs up or with one leg at a time.

4. Return to the starting position and rest with your legs extended for about 20 seconds. If you can, repeat once.

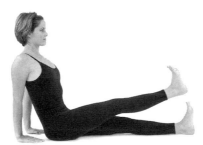

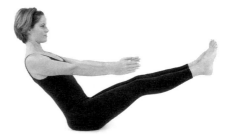

Bridge (Variation)

This posture stretches your torso, strengthens your thighs, and feels great when you've been working your abs. It is also a preparation for the Half Shoulder Stand that follows.

1. Lie on your back with your knees bent, feet on the floor at hip width. Place your arms near your sides with your palms down.
2. As you inhale, raise your hips to a comfortable height, trying to make your body a straight line from your knees to your neck. At the same time, raise your arms off the floor and bring them toward your head, without bending at the elbow. Continue the motion of your arms until your hands reach the floor behind your head, or until you need to stop.
3. As you exhale, bring your hips and arms down and return to the starting position.
4. Repeat slowly 6 to 8 times.

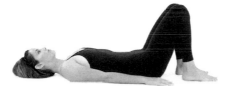

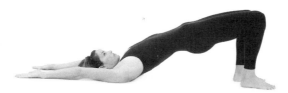

Half Shoulder Stand

Shoulder stands stimulate circulation to your head and neck and have a rejuvenating effect.

Caution: Do not use the Half Shoulder Stand if you have high blood pressure, heart disease, hiatal hernia, glaucoma, or neck problems; do not do this if you are moderately overweight or are pregnant.

1. Lie comfortably on your back, with your knees bent, feet flat on the floor, at hip width. Place your arms near your sides, palms down.

2. Exhaling, push your palms down firmly, bring your bent knees in and up, lifting your feet off the floor, straightening your legs as you raise your hips. Lift your hips off the floor as high as you comfortably can.

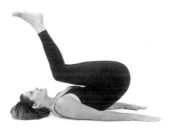

3. Continue exhaling and bend your elbows. Bring your hands to meet the top of your hips, then slide them up to your lower back. Use your elbows and the backs of your upper arms against the floor for support. Keep your legs straight but not locked, with your feet directly above your head. Try to relax your neck. Your weight will be distributed between your shoulders and your elbows, and you may have a sensation of blood flowing into your face or head.

4. When you feel ready to come down, lower your hips to the floor with the support of your hands, and then bend your knees and lower both feet to the floor.

5. Remain in the uplifted position for as long as you feel comfortable or up to 5 minutes.

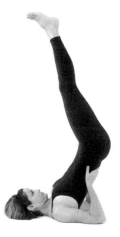

For a similar effect with less difficulty, use the supported Half Shoulder Stand, described next.

Half Shoulder Stand (Supported)
(Substitute for Half Shoulder Stand)

This posture has the same benefits as the Half Shoulder Stand, but it uses props to make it a little easier.

1. Place a bolster or several folded blankets parallel to and about 6 inches away from a wall.
2. Sit sideways on the support, and then swing your legs up the wall. Rest the back of your pelvis on the support, and rest your head, neck, and shoulders on the floor.
3. Move your buttocks toward the wall until your sit bones are relaxed in the space between the support and the wall. If you like, cover your eyes with a towel or eye bag.
4. Remain in this position for 3 to 5 minutes. When you are ready to come down, bring your knees toward your chest and slowly roll to one side.
5. Recover in the Corpse posture.

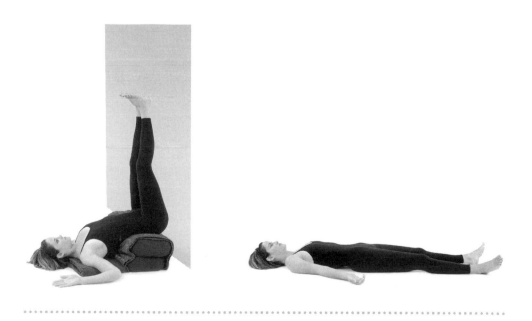

Locust (Variation)

This posture is good for general strengthening and overall stamina.

Caution: If this posture causes pain in your back or neck, leave it out.

1. Lie on your belly, with your head turned to the right, legs slightly apart with the tops of your feet on the floor.
2. Cross your hands behind your back, with your palms up, resting on your tail-bone.
3. Inhaling, raise your chest, sweep your right arm and hand forward and up, lift your left leg as high as possible, and bring your head to the middle so you are facing front.
4. Exhaling, lower your torso and leg back to the floor as you sweep your arm and hand back to your tailbone and turn your head to the left.
5. Repeat on the other side. Alternate each side 4 to 6 times.
6. To make the sequence more challenging, stay in the raised position for 4 to 6 breaths on each side after alternating 3 times on each side.

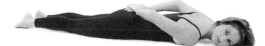

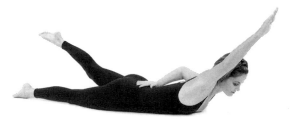

Prone Resting Posture

This is a restful posture to compensate for the strenuous Locust that preceded it.

1. Lie flat on your belly. Make a pillow with your arms and hands by bending your elbows and placing your forearms on the floor and placing your hands inward, one hand on top of the other. Turn your head to one side and rest your head on the back of your hands.
2. Stay in this position for 6 to 8 breaths.

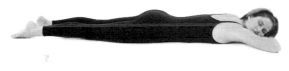

Sitting Cat

This is a very nurturing and restful posture, reminiscent of our body positioning in the womb. (If you have knee or hip problems, replace Sitting Cat with Knees to Chest, described on page 93. Thus you will be doing Knees to Chest twice in this routine.)

1. Start on your hands and knees, looking slightly down, with the heels of your hands directly below your shoulders and your knees at hip width.
2. As you exhale, sit back on your heels and bring your head toward the floor. Work toward resting your torso on your thighs with your forehead on the floor, but do not force it. Sit back only as far as comfortable.
3. Repeat 3 times, and then relax with your head down and your arms in front (as in Step 2), for 6 to 8 breaths.

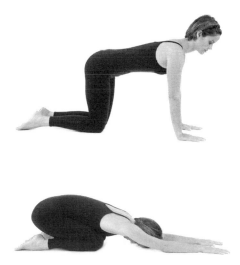

Lying Bent-Leg Twist

This is a relaxing stretch of your abs, lower back, chest, shoulders, and upper arms.

1. Lie flat on your back with your legs straight. Place your arms in a T, aligned with the tops of your shoulders, palms down.
2. Bend your right knee, bring your right foot up and place it on top of your left thigh just above the knee. Place your left hand on top of your right knee.
3. As you exhale, slowly use your left hand to press your right knee to the left toward the floor. Go as far as you can without straining. Simultaneously, turn your head to the right. You should feel the pull in your right hip.
4. Bring your right knee back upright. Lower your right knee back down to the left 3 more times. On the last time, hold the lower position for 6 to 8 breaths.
5. Return to the starting position with your legs straight.
6. Repeat the sequence with the left leg.

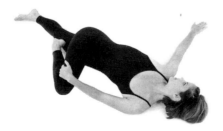

Knees to Chest

This posture relieves stiffness, misalignment, and discomfort in your lower back. We are using it to compensate for the twisting of your back in the previous posture. (Note that the Knees to Chest is different from the Knee to Chest, which appears elsewhere in the book.)

1. Lie on your back with your knees bent, feet on the floor at hip width. Bring your bent knees toward your chest and hold on to the top of your shins, just below your knees, one hand on each knee. If you are having knee problems, hold the backs of your thighs, under your knees.
2. As you exhale, draw your knees toward your chest. As you inhale, move your knees a few inches away from your chest, rolling your hips to the floor.
3. Repeat 3 times, and then stay in the most folded position for 6 to 8 breaths.
4. Remain in the Corpse position.

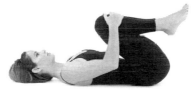

Relaxation Technique

Remain in the Corpse position. Choose one of the relaxation techniques from Chapter 5 and do it for 3 to 5 minutes.

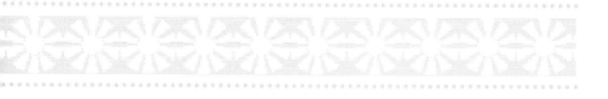

PART III

Yoga Therapy for

Common Ailments

This section is designed to help you alleviate specific health problems through carefully created Yoga routines that you can practice at home. In addition to Yoga postures, the discussion of each ailment includes nutritional and lifestyle advice that is medically sound while fitting into the overall Yoga approach to health and healing. We feel it's important that you read Chapters 1–5 and become familiar with various breathing and relaxation techniques prior to beginning any of the Yoga routines in Chapters 7–14.

If you have a serious health condition, please consult your physician for diagnosis and treatment, and mention your intent to use Yoga as a complementary therapy. Yoga may not be appropriate in the acute stage of certain ailments, such as a herniated disk or heart disease, but can be extremely beneficial in your recovery. Read the chapter carefully, and check with your health-care provider if you're not sure whether to begin Yoga therapy.

7

The Musculoskeletal System:

Back, Knees, Arthritis

arly in my career as a Yoga teacher I attended an international Yoga conference in Switzerland. Howard Kent, the founder of a British Yoga and health center, led a workshop called "The Hip Bone's Connected to the Back Bone." Illustrating with charts and diagrams, he explained the musculoskeletal system and how all its parts are tied together. Wanting us to experience the effects of that integration, he asked us to form a circle and walk around the room. After a few laps he said, "Now walk on your toes." Well, as Yoga teachers we were in good shape, but pretty soon we started to notice changes. I expected the balls of my feet to start getting tired and my toes to begin feeling numb. Beyond that, I could feel my calf muscles and knees working harder. To keep my balance, I began to lean forward and look down, thereby changing the natural curve in my back and putting it under stress. After several laps, my body was feeling strained and I had to raise my arms for balance. I looked around the room and it was quite a sight—each person's posture from head to toe was dramatically affected by walking on their toes for just ten minutes. It was a dramatic illustration of how a small alteration in our body's position can have a major effect on its overall alignment.

Your body's alignment and mobility depend on the proper relationships between elements of the musculoskeletal system—the muscles, bones, and joints. Conditions that upset the delicate balance of the musculoskeletal system often manifest as pain in your back, neck, hips, or knees. To understand why Yoga's holistic approach makes sense and how it can help, you need to know a little about the structure of your musculoskeletal system. Let's take a look at your muscles, bones, and joints and see how they respond to Yoga therapy.

ANATOMY 101

Muscles

Muscles are the body's most abundant tissue, making up about 23 percent of a woman's body and 40 percent of a man's. There are three different types of muscle in the body: cardiac muscle in the heart; smooth muscle in blood vessels and other organs; and skeletal muscle, which is the type we move voluntarily. Along with tendons and other connective tissues, the skeletal muscles provide both stability and mobility, allowing us to hold ourselves upright and to move. These are the muscles we'll be discussing here.

Skeletal muscles provide movement through contractions, working in pairs. The muscle that contracts to provide the movement is called the agonist; its opposing muscle, called the antagonist, releases and lengthens during the movement. The practice of Yoga incorporates both the contracting and the lengthening of muscles. When you hold your arms out to the sides and bend them up at the elbow (in a classic "muscle man" pose), your biceps is the agonist, contracting and shortening; and your triceps is the antagonist, stretching and lengthening. When you relax your arms, both the biceps and triceps return to their resting lengths.

When you lengthen and stretch a muscle, it opens up space for the rich flow of blood it needs to be healthy. A muscle in good condition stays relaxed at its normal resting length until needed, and it has a greater ability to produce a strong and powerful contraction. An overly stressed muscle can remain chronically tense, restricting blood supply and diminishing its strength. Yoga works primarily through gently stretching and lengthening the muscles, thereby conditioning them to be both strong and supple.

Bones and Joints

The muscles govern the movement of the skeletal system, which is composed of bones, joints, and connective tissues such as tendons, ligaments, bursae, and disks. In Yoga philosophy, joint health is a primary goal because it both influences and reflects the body's overall health.

While a few joints in the body are immovable or slightly movable, most of the joints are "freely movable" and have elaborate structures. Their complexity is one reason they're particularly vulnerable to injury.

A joint is only as healthy as the muscles surrounding it. Relaxed, flexible muscles lead to a more mobile joint. Art Brownstein, M.D., author of *Healing Back Pain Naturally,* uses the example of a stream running through the woods. Picture a tree branch jutting out from the bank of the stream into the water. At the branch, the flow of the stream is impaired and you will start to see accumulation of debris. If you remove the branch, you will see the stream quickly return to its normal speed, and it will cleanse itself of the debris that had piled up. Like the unobstructed stream, an open, limber joint has good flow and a healthy, clean surface. A major benefit of Yoga is its contribution to maintaining healthy, flexible joints.

MUSCULOSKELETAL AILMENTS

The remainder of this chapter encompasses the musculoskeletal disorders typically alleviated through Yoga therapy. Muscle, bone, and joint conditions can be caused by accident or injury, but most often they're the result of problems caused over time by such things as poor sitting posture, incorrect lifting, and even jogging on hard surfaces. Often when these problems are corrected, the corresponding pain diminishes. Many of the muscle and joint pains Westerners have come to expect as a normal part of growing older are not, in fact, inevitable and can be avoided or reversed with Yoga therapy.

Back Pain

"It's a miracle, Larry." That was music to my ears, even though it was fifteen years after I had treated Robert, a respected screenwriter in Hollywood. He had come to me in desperation, a last-ditch effort to avoid surgery on his chronically aching back. Having seen every specialist in town from orthopedists to chiropractors, he was out of options and still suffering. His diagnosis was "a posterior bulging disk between L4 and L5." In English, an intervertebral disk (a jelly-doughnut-like pad) in his lower back was bulging backward out of its normal position. It appeared that the pressure of the bulging disk on the nerves was causing pain and numbness in his back and down his right leg. I spoke to his orthopedic doctor, reviewed his diagnosis, and got the go-ahead to begin Yoga therapy. (Depending on the disk problem, certain types of bending and twisting can cause further damage. A regular group Yoga class, in which individual instruction is usually minimal, would have been a big mistake.)

Our one-on-one Yoga therapy treatments began with Yoga breathing to relax the back muscles. I added simple breath and movement patterns, avoiding forward bends and emphasizing gentle arching postures. We discussed his lifestyle, and he admitted spending hours at the computer in a slumped forward position. It was easy to adjust the level of his computer screen so his spine would be upright. The results were stunning. His pain quickly subsided as he responded to the treatment while diligently practicing his Yoga therapy routine twice a day.

After a few short months, Robert was able to attend my group class. He knew what to avoid and how to modify postures to fit his condition. Because he lived on the other side of town, he found a good Yoga center near him, and eventually I lost track of him. Years later, walking through the health club, I heard my name called. Grinning and shaking my hand, Robert told me he'd joined a weekly Yoga class and kept up with it, and his back pain had never returned. Even after all these years, he couldn't conceal his enthusiasm as he admitted he'd thought relief from back pain was an impossible dream.

Most people experience back pain at some point in their lives, and many miss work or even become disabled because of it. Perhaps 90 percent of people with acute back pain get better within a month. While for a number of people the pain subsides within a few months, others develop chronic back pain that persists for months or even years. This is the type of pain most likely to be relieved by Yoga therapy. If you suffer from back pain, be sure to read the Yoga Prescription for Musculoskeletal Ailments on page 111 and Yoga for the Back on page 114.

When we think of the back, we usually think first of the spine—a partially flexible column of bones and disks that extends from the base of the skull to the pelvis. It provides the torso's vertical support, and transfers the weight of the upper body through the pelvis and down to the feet. The spine also encloses and protects the spinal cord, a bundle of nerves connecting every area of the body to the brain. The spinal column is uniquely constructed to guard the spinal cord while also providing strong but flexible upper body support.

The spine is made up of vertebrae and their joints, each of which can move in six different directions. (That's a lot of movable parts, increasing the odds of something going wrong.) The vertebrae are bound together by two long, thick ligaments running the entire length of the spine as well as by smaller ligaments between each pair of vertebrae.

The uppermost section of the spine, the seven vertebrae of the neck, is known as the cervical spine. The middle section, made up of twelve vertebrae, is called the thoracic spine, which is the longest section of spine. The lower section is called the lumbar spine, which is the inward-curving small of the back that is made up of five vertebrae. The sacrum is both the base of the spine and the back of the pelvis. As the foundation of the higher levels of the spine, the position of the sacrum plays an important role in the overall alignment of your back. Tip the sacrum too far forward for too long, for example, and the curvature of the whole spine gets distorted and sends you running to your local Yoga therapist.

You might think of the spine as running in a straight line down the middle of the back, but only if viewed from directly behind. Seen from the side, the spine is curved, with each spinal section having its own characteristic curve: the cervical (neck) and the lumbar each curve toward the inside of the body, and the thoracic and the sacral each curve toward the outside (Figure 1).

The spinal curves are important to the structure of the body, acting as a kind of shock absorber and a bal-

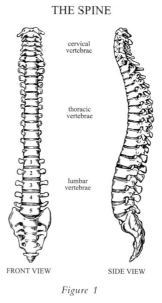

THE SPINE

cervical vertebrae

thoracic vertebrae

lumbar vertebrae

FRONT VIEW   SIDE VIEW

Figure 1

ancing mechanism for the torso. Distorting the curves, either by increasing or decreasing them, can have negative effects for our overall health. Since the back's proper alignment is paramount, one of the primary goals of Yoga therapy is to restore and preserve the proper curvature of the spine.

The back also consists of a complex musculature, which is tied in with the muscles in your head, arms, and legs. Different muscles in the back can be affected by muscles in other parts of the body. For example, the hamstrings (the back of the thighs) pull on the bottom of the pelvis in a way that tends to affect the lumbar region of the spine. If your hamstrings are tight, they can exert such a tremendous pressure on your spine that they can literally flatten the normal lumbar curve. People with occupations that involve sitting in one position for long periods of time, especially taxi and truck drivers, often have back pain that can be helped by loosening up the hamstrings.

While most back problems are musculoskeletal (related to muscles, bones and joints, tendons and ligaments), back pain can also be caused by kidney infections, ulcers, gastrointestinal distress, reproductive organ problems, other internal organ disorders, and even cancer. **For this reason, if you experience severe or persistent back pain, it is imperative to receive a diagnosis from a physician.** If tests have confirmed that your back pain is not caused by an underlying organ problem or disease and you are not in an acute stage of pain, then starting with a Yoga therapy program is appropriate and will most likely bring relief.

By far the most common back pain is lower back strain. The pain may start suddenly after heavy lifting or twisting, but the structural weakness was most likely set in place long before, through your patterns of movement or as a result of an accident or injury. Women may first notice back pain in pregnancy, and dads can feel lower back strain after carrying their children. If you sit at a desk for long hours leaning forward toward a computer, if you often wear high heels, or if your job involves heavy lifting, you're a prime candidate for lower back strain.

Herb was a retired seventy-three-year-old movie producer and pianist who had suffered from serious lower back problems and terrible posture since adolescence. As he aged, his back pain worsened, but he had found no relief through traditional medical channels. Easily the stiffest man I had ever treated, Herb had compounded his back problems by playing the piano with poor posture for years. I started by giving him routines specifically targeted for back and neck problems.

He was diligent about his daily Yoga practice, and as his symptoms gradually improved, I updated his program to keep up with his progress. Within six months, Herb was engaging in a daily one-hour program and was symptom free after more than fifty years of chronic back problems.

While acute back pain usually heals within a month or two, chronic back pain is less responsive to medical and chiropractic solutions. The good news is that chronic low back pain can usually be managed or eliminated by regular practice of simple Yoga therapy techniques, such as in the Lower Back Routine outlined in this chapter.

Another type of back pain is the result of damaged disks. A normal, healthy spine has a wide range of motion, and the intervertebral disks play a big part in this extraordinary flexibility (Figure 2). You know those jelly-filled doughnuts we're not supposed to eat because they're so fattening? They look a little bit like our intervertebral disks. Made of a tough outer ring that surrounds a gel-filled pocket, a disk is positioned between each pair of vertebrae in your spine. Like little shock

THE INTERVERTEBRAL DISK

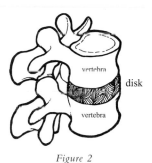

Figure 2

absorbers, they cushion the vertebrae and soften the forces created by movement such as walking and jumping. You may have heard the term "slipped disk," layperson's language for what's technically called a herniated disk. The disk doesn't really slip, but its outer ring gives way so that the gel inside bulges out from between the vertebrae and can press against the spinal nerves.

Disk problems usually cause acute pain and require medical attention. Symptoms of disk disorders commonly include numbness or tingling sensations in the legs and feet, or sharp, immobilizing pains in the back. **Note: If you have a disk problem, or if you haven't obtained a diagnosis but you have these symptoms, be sure to consult a physician before starting any Yoga practice.** If you have acute pain, begin Yoga only with your doctor's approval.

Most disk problems heal on their own over time; however, the pain may be so debilitating or long lasting that your doctor may suggest surgery. Unfortunately, there is no guarantee that back surgery will eliminate the pain. Yoga therapy can be helpful with many disk problems after the acute stage has passed, as long as your doctor feels the movement will not exacerbate your condition. If your doctor approves, follow either the upper- or the lower-back routines described in this chapter, depending on the location of your pain. Remember, if any of the movements increase your pain—stop. Practice only those postures that enhance your feeling of well-being, and do them gently.

Another common contributor to back pain is stress. Many of us are familiar with that tight, tension-filled ache in the neck or shoulders that just yearns to be rubbed or dunked in a hot tub. And someone suffering from undue stress might bend over to pick something up and develop a back muscle spasm, and not be able to get up. Many studies have been performed to investigate the powerful mind–body connection, confirming that our mental stress does influence our muscles.

If you've been in a car accident or suffered an activity-related injury, your back may be feeling the pain for months or even years afterward. Sometimes the pain leads to dysfunctional movement patterns—that is, you compensate for the pain by adjusting your sitting, standing, or walking posture. This puts your body even further out of balance and can lead to other problems in your back, neck, or hips. The tension in the injured area may leave it feeling chronically "tight" and lacking flexibility. The tightness may interfere with healing by preventing good circulation in the injured area. Since Yoga therapy addresses these problems, it can be a great help in treating injury-related back pain. A carefully practiced Yoga therapy routine, such as the back routines given in this chapter, can help or even completely alleviate the back pain. Your Yoga practice may also help you correct any dysfunctional movement patterns or postures you have developed, a crucial step toward healing.

Knees

Of all the joints in your body, your knees may be the most susceptible to pain or injury. Our knees are subject to numerous stresses as we go about our daily lives, walking, lifting, and kneeling. When we go all-out in high-impact activities such as jogging, skiing, or playing basketball, we're asking our knees to perform above and beyond the call of duty, especially when we twist and turn, stop and start, or jump. Pain in the knee is usually a direct result of these daily and extraordinary stresses, either from an injury or simply from excessive wear and tear over time.

Cartilage is found in the knee in three places: under the kneecap, on the ends of the femur and tibia, and in the joint itself. Abnormal wearing of the cartilage can be caused by trauma or overuse of the knee. Cartilage can be torn by forcefully rotating the knee beyond its endurance. Pain can vary from mild to severe, and there may be swelling.

When the tendons are injured and become inflamed, it is known as tendinitis, which can be quite painful. It is usually caused by a repetitive motion that over-stresses the tendon; "tennis elbow" results from the repeated swing of the tennis racket over weeks, months, or years. Tendinitis of the knee is sometimes referred to as "jumper's knee," since the high impact of jumping strains the tendons. Pain is usually mild during normal activity but severe when the tendon is being overused, such as in high-impact aerobics or running. The extreme version of tendinitis is a ruptured or torn tendon, which most often occurs in older people whose tendons are weaker and less elastic. When this happens in the knee, it's quite painful and makes bending or extending the leg difficult.

Car accidents and contact sports are often responsible for ligament injury, when there is a direct blow to the knee area. These injuries are also commonly caused by sudden twisting motions, as in the quick stop–start of basketball. Ligament sprains, strains, or tears usually cause pain, swelling, and difficulty walking; often, the knee will buckle and there will be a popping sensation.

When the cartilage of the knee degenerates and gradually wears away, it is known as osteoarthritis. It's usually caused by excess stress on the joint over an extended period. (Be sure to read the more detailed explanation of arthritis in the next section.)

Because knee ailments and patients vary so much, so do their treatments. Your physician will make decisions on how to treat your knee based on the exact nature of the injury or condition, the severity of it, your health history, and your personal preference. Treatments for knee injuries can involve pain medication, physical therapy, exercise programs, applying ice, wearing a brace, limiting activity, or any combination of these. If your knee condition is severe, your doctor may recommend surgery.

The Yoga therapy routine for knees in this chapter is an excellent tool for recovery from a knee injury or disease, and it may be especially effective in rehabilitation from knee surgery to begin restoring flexibility to the joint and strength to the muscles. Be sure to work in conjunction with your physician and/or physical therapist to maximize your healing and avoid further injury.

If you normally approach exercise and sports with the "no pain-no gain" attitude, you might as well drop it right now. It's not going to help you, especially when you're dealing with a joint as vulnerable as the knee. I know all too well what can happen when we Westerners insist on tackling Yoga with a "just do it" mentality.

Twenty years ago, I took a month-long Yoga teacher training course at a remote ashram in southern India. The courses and meals were taught and served on the floor. One of the goals was to sit in the full lotus posture as much as possible, which was very easy for the Indians. Yoga postures were developed in India for people who traditionally used very little furniture, squatted daily for numerous reasons, and kept their knee and hip joints very limber. However, for a mid-thirties, ex-jock male from California, a comfortable lotus position is more of a two-year plan than a thirty-day intensive. Unfortunately, I let my competitive spirit get the best of me. One morning during meditation, I finally twisted my legs far enough to sit very painfully in the full lotus posture. Exuberant because I had reached "the goal," I ignored the warning signs coming from my knee joints and eventually felt a deep burning in my right knee. After another few minutes I also felt a tearing sensation. I knew something was wrong, but didn't realize until I returned to the United States that I had torn the cartilage in my right knee. I tried for two years to fix it through Yoga and physical therapy but finally had to resort to arthroscopic surgery. Eventually, I was able to use Yoga therapy to assist in my post-op healing, and I've kept my knees healthy ever since.

The point to remember is that the Yoga perspective never involves increasing the pain as a means to an end. As you begin to apply Yoga therapy for recovery from your painful knee, listen to your body. Challenge but don't strain yourself. Don't push yourself into any Yoga posture that causes or increases pain.

If you're suffering from pain in your knees, it is crucial that you see a physician for diagnosis and treatment. People often seek help from a Yoga teacher or therapist when the pain first hits, but the time for Yoga therapy is not in the acute stage, which usually involves severe pain and inflammation. Once you are on the road to recovery and you want to enhance your body's healing process, you should get your doctor's okay before starting a Yoga therapy program. If you suffer from a painful knee, be sure to read the Yoga Prescription for Musculoskeletal Ailments on page 111.

Arthritis

Turn on the television any day of the week and you'll be bombarded by commercials aimed at arthritis sufferers. The message is that arthritis equals pain—pain that keeps us from playing the piano, enjoying a round of golf, or holding our grandchildren. Arthritis is so common in our culture that most people, including doctors, have come to accept it as a natural part of growing older. Even though arthritis is not life-threatening, it can steal away your quality of life, forcing you to limit or stop not only the physical activities you enjoy but those you need to get you through the day—like walking, dressing, and cooking.

About forty-two million Americans—nearly 20 percent of our population—suffer from some form of arthritis. A whopping 85 percent of people over age sixty-five show evidence of arthritis on x-ray, and half of those experience symptoms.[1] It has a huge impact on work and is second only to heart disease as a reason that people leave employment.

Arthritis has everything to do with movement, which is one reason Yoga therapy can be particularly effective for helping it. If you have arthritis, you may be so sore that you curtail your movements. When you don't move enough, your joints freeze up and become stiff, which increases the pain, making you even less likely to move. It's a vicious circle, and the longer it continues, the more functions you may lose. Movement also can be one of the causes of arthritis, particularly stressful or destructive movement patterns over time, and the pain of arthritis can be assuaged through the right kind of movement.

The word *arthritis* means "joint inflammation," and there are more than one hundred arthritic diseases, each causing pain, swelling, and stiffness in the joints. The most common type is osteoarthritis. It's sometimes called degenerative joint disease, or wear-and-tear arthritis.

Osteoarthritis means that the joints have worn down over time. Repetitive overuse or injury causes cartilage to be destroyed, leaving the ends of the bone unprotected. The joint then loses mobility and becomes painful. You can get osteoarthritis in the joints of your fingers, feet, hips, knees, or spine; but it's improbable you'd have it in your wrist, elbows, shoulders, or jaw. Arthritic symptoms in these areas are more likely another arthritic condition such as rheumatoid arthritis.

Rheumatoid, or inflammatory, arthritis is the second most common type of arthritis. An autoimmune disorder causes your own antibodies to attack perfectly healthy joint tissues, causing extreme swelling, pain, and redness. The inflammation can jump like fire from one joint to the next, and even into organs. Unlike osteoarthritis, it causes pain and swelling in many joints and locations, not just a specific area. The inflammation is extremely painful and leads to permanent joint damage.

But arthritis affects more than just your joints—your muscles take a hit, too. The National Arthritis Foundation has determined from multiple research projects that much of the pain in a severely arthritic joint is from the muscles, not from inside the joint. Dr. Art Brownstein likens it to putting a cast on a completely healthy arm and leaving it on for a year. When you take the cast off, your arm would be rigid and sore, not because of the joints but because the muscles have atrophied. They'd be weaker, thinner, shorter, tighter, and stiffer. It would become very painful to use them. Similarly, arthritis makes you behave as if your limbs are in a cast unable to move, leading to atrophy, so the aching joint is compounded by aching muscles. Relief is impossible without proper exercise to move the joints and rebuild the muscles. If you have your arthritic knee replaced with a shiny new titanium model but you don't begin a regular stretching and exercise program, eventually your pain will be the same as it was before the surgery, because of those atrophied muscles.

Just because you have achy joints, don't assume you have arthritis. Overuse injuries can result in other conditions such as tendinitis, bursitis, or carpal tunnel syndrome. As always, get diagnosed by a physician before jumping to conclusions.

Of all the testimonials in this book, the one closest to my heart is from my own brother. Harold Payne is a well-traveled performing songwriter with extensive credits including more than hundred recordings by artists ranging from Patti LaBelle to Rod Stewart to long time collaborator, Bobby Womack. At age thirty-nine, Harold was diagnosed with ankylosing spondylitis (AS), a severe form of inflammatory arthritis with no cure. AS affects the spine by attacking the joints, eventually fusing them. It is sometimes referred to as "bamboo spine" and can also affect other joints, such as the shoulders, hips, knees, and feet.

Harold decided to use every resource possible to make the best of the situation. He tried chiropractic treatments, physical therapy, and water exercise in addition to regular Yoga therapy sessions with me and world-renowned Yoga master T. K. V. Desikachar. Under the guidance of a rheumatologist, Harold took nonsteroidal anti-inflammatory drugs (NSAIDs) to reduce pain and suppress inflammation. Another important factor was education from the Spondylitis Association of America.

As a result of his holistic *Yoga Rx* approach, sixteen years after diagnosis Harold is a role model for AS. He stands tall with good posture, does not need medication, and participates in regular group Yoga classes. He continues to travel and perform internationally and believes his positive attitude despite the illness has had a major impact on his health.

The bottom line on arthritis is that there is no cure. Once the disease gets started, nobody is sure whether it can be completely stopped in its tracks. However, contemporary scientific research and ancient Yoga philosophy both agree it's possible to slow it down and to ease symptoms enough to bring back your enjoyment of life. For an excellent in-depth resource, I recommend the book *Preventing Arthritis* by Ron Lawrence, M.D., Ph.D., and Martin Zucker. If you suffer from arthritis, be sure to read the Yoga Prescription for Musculoskeletal Ailments on page 111, and Yoga for Arthritis on page 145.

The Yoga Advantage for Musculoskeletal Ailments

Both of the authors of this book were introduced to Yoga because of serious, long-term musculoskeletal pain. We tried numerous remedies without success and finally found lasting relief through Yoga therapy. We're each aware of many others with the same experience. So in our opinion, Yoga practiced properly and consistently is one of the best ways, if not *the* best way, to manage pain in your muscles, bones, and joints.

The benefits of Yoga for these ailments are numerous and in many ways unique among all types of exercise. The routines given in this chapter will relax your entire body with Yoga breathing and create a union of your body, breath, and mind. You will gently stretch and strengthen your muscles without worsening any existing pain. The asymmetrical postures will stretch each side of your body area separately, important because the strength and flexibility of the muscles on either side of the body are frequently uneven from long-term unequal use. Yoga promotes circulation to the injured area, while strengthening the muscles and loosening up chronic painful contractions.

The Yoga therapy routines in this chapter are designed not only to enhance the health of your muscles but also to improve the condition of your joints. Unlike other exercises that may continue to stress your joints, in Yoga you move slowly and gently, practicing postures that gently pull the joint surfaces apart. This is followed by postures that stretch and strengthen the surrounding muscles to support the joint. Yoga also works to correct improper movement patterns that may be causing joint pain, through repetition of the Yoga routine to establish a more healthy range of motion. The combination of stretching, strengthening, and correcting movement patterns increases joint flexibility, supporting healing and allowing pain to diminish.

Since many of us are at risk for muscle and joint problems at some point in our lives, the Yoga routines in this chapter can be used preventatively. We especially encourage "weekend warrior" type athletes to practice the routines to reduce the risk of injury from tight muscles and unhealthy joints. People with osteoporosis can improve their balance and overall strength by practicing these routines, to reduce their risk of falls that can lead to bone fracture and subsequent debilitating pain.

While the positive effects of exercise on joint problems have been accepted in the Yoga culture for centuries, the idea is fairly new in the scientific community. Recently, researchers at Philadelphia's Hahnemann University and the University of Pennsylvania School of Medicine presented a paper suggesting that correctly performed Yoga may actually alter cells and protect cartilage tissue, preserving the function of joints.[2] Various studies are under way to explore the medical basis for the link between Yoga and joint health.

In years gone by, if you had a knee or back ailment you were given strict instructions to stay off of it. But evidence since the 1980s has turned that advice on its head, with study after study proving that musculoskeletal ailments only get worse with inactivity. So now the old axiom "use it or lose it" is applied to most knee and back problems, and is especially true for those who have arthritis.

Numerous studies have now shown that the best way to prevent and treat arthritis is to keep moving. The U.S. Centers for Disease Control and Prevention released a report to counter mistaken recommendations in the past that persons with arthritis should not exercise because it would damage their joints.[3] Most physicians recommend a program of flexibility, strengthening, and endurance exercises, which together can improve your general sense of well-being, decrease pain, and possibly even slow the arthritic process. Yoga therapy is uniquely effective for recovery from joint problems because if you do it according to the instructions, there is no bouncing, no impact, and no pushing yourself beyond your limits. Yoga provides exactly the kind of movement an arthritic joint needs, and if your arthritis is severe, Yoga might be about the only exercise you feel you can do.

Yoga has another advantage specifically for rheumatoid arthritis, in that this disease appears to be worsened by stress. Several studies have shown that a program of exercise and stress reduction can greatly reduce the flare-ups of rheumatoid arthritis. A major study published in *Rheumatic Disease Clinics of North America* suggested that therapies focusing on calming the mind, relaxing the body, and improving general health considerably reduced patients' pain and may have even promoted healing of the arthritis.[4]

While there are reams of anecdotal evidence establishing the effectiveness of Yoga for musculoskeletal pain, a landmark paper titled "Asana Based Exercises for the Management of Low Back Pain" was the first to scientifically support it.[5] Conducted at the Indian Institute of Technology, the study involved patients with lower back pain who were given a series of Yoga postures to perform regularly. After six months, 70 percent of the participants reported significant improvement, with near normal mobility and absence of pain. Those whose back pain continued also admitted they had not practiced the Yoga regularly.[6] The results of this study perfectly mirror our experience with patients suffering musculoskeletal pain: When they commit to a regular Yoga therapy practice, most find relief fairly quickly. If you apply Yoga's holistic approach, looking at all the factors in your life that could be contributing to your pain, you may find that your ailments will heal themselves better than you ever thought possible.

The Yoga Prescription for Musculoskeletal Ailments

❋ Develop a regular exercise program for overall fitness and cardiovascular conditioning. Avoid activities that cause intense pain.

* Swimming or exercising in the water is an excellent way to complement your Yoga therapy routine. It will strengthen your muscles and keep you flexible, without putting pressure on your joints. An excellent resource for water exercise is *The Water Power Workout* by Robert Forster, P.T., and Lynda Huey, M.A.

* Cycling and walking are also good forms of low-impact cardiovascular exercise.

* To avoid stress on your joints, aim for short but frequent exercise sessions.

* Look at your patterns of moving and carrying. Be creative in finding ways to reduce stress on your back and your knee and hip joints: Use your legs when picking things up, use carts with wheels when possible, carry lighter loads, or simply get someone else to do the heavy lifting.

* Take frequent breaks in repetitive motion.

* Decrease your sedentary time. If you are required to sit at a desk for many hours, take breaks at least once an hour to walk around. Instead of watching television in the evening, try taking a walk (as your pain allows).

* If you're overweight, losing just ten pounds can significantly reduce the strain on your knees and back, relieving arthritis and other types of pain.

* Eat a wholesome diet to increase your general sense of well-being, making sure to get plenty of calcium for healthy bones. You can get enough calcium by taking a supplement or including in your diet calcium-rich foods, such as dairy products, salmon, and dark green leafy vegetables.

* Keep in mind that Yoga therapy is best once you're out of the acute stage of pain. The Yoga routines in this chapter are excellent for chronic musculoskeletal pain problems and rehabilitation from surgery or an acute episode.

* Talk to your doctor about using pain relievers and/or nonsteroidal anti-inflammatory drugs such as ibuprofen and acetaminophen.

* Make a serious effort to reduce the mental stress in your life, which often shows up as pain in your back or neck and which can exacerbate arthritis. Doing Yoga is a stress buster.

- Wear low-heeled shoes that fit properly and give good support to help maintain your balance and leg alignment.
- Glucosamine and chondroitin sulfate have been in the news lately, being touted as arthritis remedies. Each is a natural substance found in and around cartilage. If you are diabetic or obese, you should stay away from glucosamine. We recommend you discuss with your doctor whether these supplements are appropriate for you.
- Capsaicin, a component of red hot peppers, has been shown to provide arthritis pain relief when applied as a skin preparation. It appears to do more than just mask the pain, providing long-term relief from pain when used regularly. It is available in over-the-counter preparations, but should be used with extreme caution because even a miniscule amount in your eyes can cause severe burning and irritation.
- Approach Yoga and any other exercise slowly, especially when joints are stiff or muscles are tight. Being too aggressive can make it worse.
- Practice the appropriate Yoga therapy routine from this chapter. Start with two or three days a week, working toward five to six days a week.

Yoga for the Back

Lower Back Routine

The following is a program for lower back strain, or for the rehabilitation of chronic back pain, similar to the one I devised for Herb (page 102). When you begin, do only Phase One postures, those marked with an arrow (⇾), for two to four weeks. This will take about twenty minutes. When you are ready for Phase Two, use all of the postures in the order they are presented. Phase Two will take about thirty minutes. Use Belly Breathing (page 41) or Focused Breathing (page 39) throughout. As you become more comfortable, you can incorporate the more advanced breathing technique called Victorious Breath (page 44). Ideally, practice the routine twice a day until your condition improves, then practice it once a day. When you feel your condition has subsided, you may cut down to three times a week.

Caution: This routine is not for anyone in acute or severe pain. If your pain is accompanied by other symptoms, such as numbness or weakness in your legs, it is advisable to check with your doctor before using this program.

. . . .

⇾ *Bent-Legs Corpse* ⇽

This is the classic posture for relaxation of the mind–body. Bending your legs supports your back.

1. Lie on your back with your arms at your sides, palms up.
2. Bend your knees with your feet on the floor at hip width. If your head tilts back or if your neck or throat is tense, use a pillow or folded blanket under your head. Stay in the posture for 8 to 10 breaths.
3. Relax with your eyes closed.

. . . .

→ *Knee to Chest* ←

This easy stretch relieves stiffness, misalignment, and discomfort in the lower back. You can also use it for compensation after back bends and twists. (Note: Knee to Chest is different from Knees to Chest, which appears elsewhere in the book.)

1. Lie on your back, with your knees bent and feet on the floor at hip width.
2. As you exhale, draw the right knee into the chest. Hold your shin just below your knee. If you have knee problems, hold the back of your thigh near your knee.
3. If it feels comfortable, slide your left foot and leg down slowly to their full extended position on the floor, keeping your right knee at your chest. If this causes discomfort, bring your left leg back into the bent-knee position.
4. Stay in this posture for 6 to 8 breaths. Bring both legs back to the bent-knee position.
5. Then repeat on your left side.

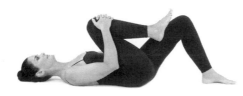

→ *Lying Arm Raise with Bent Leg* ←

This simple arm movement gently stretches the muscles of the upper and lower back, working each side of the back separately, since so many back problems are asymmetrical, or one sided. It also promotes circulation to your neck and shoulders.

1. Lie flat on your back with your arms at your sides, palms down. Bend your right knee and place your right foot on the floor.
2. As you inhale, slowly raise both arms up and overhead touching the floor behind you, palms up. Pause briefly.
3. Exhaling, bring your arms back to your sides.
4. Repeat the arm raise 4 to 6 times. Then lower your right leg.
5. Bring your left leg to the bent knee position. Repeat the arm raise 4 to 6 times.

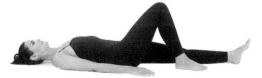

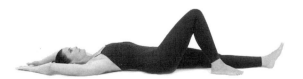

→ *Push Downs* ←

This exercise strengthens your entire abdomen, focusing on your lower abdomen below the navel.

1. Lie on your back with bent knees, feet on the floor at hip width. Place your arms at your sides, palms down.
2. Take a deep breath, and as you exhale, slowly push your lower back down into the floor for 5 to 7 seconds. You should feel your lower abs contracting and the curve of your lower back flattening.
3. As you inhale, release your back.
4. Repeat 6 to 8 times.

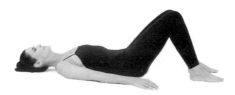

Yoga Crunches

In these crunches, the emphasis is on slow, controlled movement. They strengthen and tone the abdomen, especially the upper abs above the navel. They also strengthen the inside of the thighs (adductors), the neck, and the shoulders.

1. Lie on your back, bend your knees, and place your feet on the floor at hip width.
2. Turn your heels out and toes in (pigeon-toed). Tilt your inner knees together until they touch.
3. Interlace your fingers behind your head, and hook your thumbs under the angle of the jawbone, slightly below the ears.
4. As you exhale, push your knees together firmly, tilt your pelvis toward your navel, and use your abdominal muscles to slowly sit up, keeping your hips on the floor. Go only halfway up, so that about half your back is off the floor. Keep your elbows wide and to the sides, in alignment with the tops of your shoulders, using your hands to support your head. Look toward the tops of your knees. Do not pull your head up with your arms.
5. As you inhale, slowly roll back down.
6. Repeat 6 to 8 times.

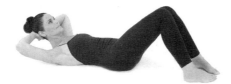

✤ *Bridge* ✦

This posture can be used for compensation after abdominal exercises. It promotes circulation to the neck and the shoulders while strengthening and stretching the back, shoulders, hips, and thighs.

1. Lie on your back, bend your knees, and place your feet on the floor at hip width.
2. Relax your arms at your sides, palms down.
3. As you inhale, use your abdominal muscles to raise your hips halfway up. Pause. Then lift your hips as high as you feel comfortable. Do not go past halfway if it causes you any back pain.
4. As you exhale, bring your hips back to the floor.
5. Repeat 6 to 8 times, remembering to pause halfway up.

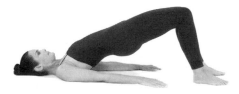

⇥ *Bent-Leg Hamstring Stretch* ⇤

This stretch feels great on the hamstrings, and prepares the body for numerous sitting, kneeling, and standing postures.

1. Lie on your back with your knees bent, feet on the floor at hip width. Relax your arms at your sides, palms down.
2. As you exhale, bring your right knee toward your chest, and hold the back of the right thigh with both hands just below your knee.
3. As you inhale, extend your right leg up toward the ceiling, as high as feels comfortable. Do not force it—your leg does not need to be fully locked out. Keep your foot flexed. Bring your entire leg as close to your head as you can.
4. As you exhale, return your leg to the bent position, but don't return your foot to the floor. Keep your head and the top of your hips on the floor. If the back of your head tilts back or your throat tenses while raising or lowering the leg, place a pillow or blanket under your head.
5. Repeat the leg extension 3 to 4 times. Then hold the extended leg with your hands interlaced on the back of the thigh for 6 to 8 breaths.
6. Return both legs to bent-knee position with your feet on the floor. Repeat the entire sequence using your left leg.

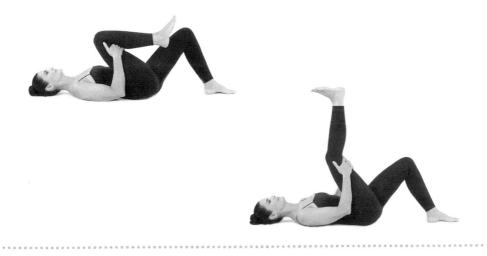

Balancing Cat

This posture helps improve your overall balance and stability.

1. Start on your hands and knees with the heels of your hands directly below your shoulders, your knees at hip width.
2. As you exhale, slowly slide your right hand forward and your left leg backward as far as they will go on the ground. Pause briefly.
3. As you inhale, raise your right hand and left leg up as high as you feel comfortable or until they are both parallel to the floor. As you exhale, bring them both down to the floor, keeping them in the extended position.
4. Repeat the lifting motion 3 times, then hold in the lifted position for 4 to 6 breaths.
5. Repeat the sequence with your left arm and right leg. Return to the starting position on your hands and knees.

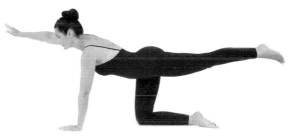

Sitting Cat

This is a gentle stretch for your lower back, helping it relax and loosen up any tension. It is often used as a compensation posture after back bends or back stretches, which is how it's being used here.

1. Start on your hands and knees with the heels of your hands directly below your shoulders and your knees at hip width. Look down slightly.
2. As you exhale, sit back on your heels. Relax in the posture and try to rest your torso on your thighs and your forehead on the floor. Do not force yourself beyond your comfort zone.
3. Repeat 3 times, then relax with your head down and arms in front (as in Step 2) for 6 to 8 breaths.

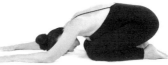

→ *Cobra* ←

The Cobra increases flexibility to the lower back and strengthens the arms, chest, and shoulders. It opens the chest to promote a deeper breathing pattern.

Caution: If the Cobra causes any pain or discomfort, replace it with the Sphinx (described next). If both postures cause discomfort, leave them out.

1. Lie flat on your belly, legs at hip width, with the front of your feet on the floor. If you have lower back problems, it is important to separate your legs slightly wider than your hips and to turn your heels out.
2. Rest your forehead on the floor and relax your shoulders. Place your palms on the floor with your thumbs near your armpits and your fingers facing forward. Your elbows should be bent close to your sides.
3. Inhaling, engage your back muscles, push your palms down against the floor, and lift your chest and head, looking straight ahead. Leave the front of the pelvis on the floor and keep your shoulders dropped and relaxed. Push yourself as high as feels comfortable, keeping your elbows bent, unless your back is very flexible. To make this easier, move your hands farther forward. To make it more challenging, move your hands farther back.
4. Exhaling, lower your torso and head slowly back to the ground.
5. Repeat the lift 6 to 8 times.

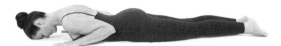

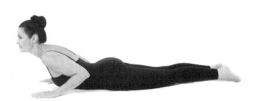

→ *Sphinx (Substitute for Cobra)* ←

Use the Sphinx if you are not ready for the Cobra. The Sphinx emphasizes flexibility of the upper back and strengthens the arms, chest, and shoulders. It opens the chest, promoting a deeper breathing pattern.

1. Lie flat on your belly, legs at hip width, tops of your feet on the floor.
2. Relax your forehead on the floor and release your shoulders. Place your forearms on the floor, palms turned down, near the sides of your head.
3. As you inhale, push your forearms against the floor, and lift your chest and head. Look forward and straight ahead. Your forearms and the front of your pelvis should stay on the floor. Try to keep your shoulders relaxed.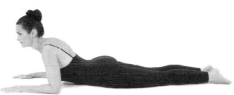
4. As you exhale, slowly lower yourself down to the floor.
5. Repeat the lift 6 to 8 times.

Prone Resting Posture

This is a relaxing posture, similar to the Corpse. Use it to rest your back after doing prone (lying on the belly) back bends like the Cobra or Sphinx.

1. Lie on your belly, legs at hip width with the front of your feet on the floor.
2. Gently place your forehead on the floor or turn your head to one side. Bend your elbows, and rest your forearms on the floor. Turn your palms down, and place them near the sides of your head.
3. Hold the posture for 6 to 8 breaths.

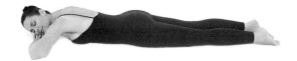

Locust (Supported)

This posture strengthens the entire trunk, including the lower and upper back, neck, arms, shoulders, buttocks, and legs. It also helps build overall stamina.

Caution: Be careful not to strain your back when doing this posture. If necessary, use the options in Step 3 to make it less strenuous.

1. Lie flat on your belly with a folded blanket under your hips. Place your legs at hip width with the front of your feet on the floor. Rest your forehead on the floor.
2. Rest your arms on the floor along the sides of your body, palms down.
3. Inhaling, raise your chest, head, and right leg. If the pose is too strenuous, try just bending the leg at the knee. For an even easier variation, raise the chest without lifting the leg at all. To make the posture more challenging, raise both legs.
4. As you exhale, lower your trunk, head, and leg slowly to the floor.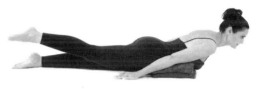
5. Repeat the lift 6 to 8 times.
6. Repeat with your left leg.

⇥ Sitting Cat ⇤

Repeating this gentle stretch for the lower back will help it relax and loosen up any tension. (If you have knee or hip problems, replace the Sitting Cat with the Knees to Chest, described on page 126.)

1. Start on your hands and knees, looking slightly down, with the heels of your hands directly below your shoulders and your knees at hip width.
2. As you exhale, sit back on your heels and bring your head toward the floor. Work toward resting your torso on your thighs with your forehead on the floor, but do not force it. Only sit back as far as comfortable.
3. Repeat 3 times and then relax in the posture with your arms in front, for 6 to 8 breaths.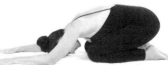

✧ *Lying Bent-Legs Twist* ✧

This gentle twisting motion promotes circulation to your back. It tones the abdomen and usually feels great to those of us with stiff backs.

Caution: Move carefully and slowly while executing a twist. If you experience any pain or discomfort, leave the twist out of your routine until you can check with your health professional.

1. Lie flat on your back, knees bent, feet on the floor at hip width. Place your arms straight out from your sides in a T, palms down, level with your shoulders.
2. Exhale and slowly lower your bent legs to the right side, turning your head to the left. Your shoulders and head remain flat on the floor, but your left hip will come off the floor. While in this position, your entire right leg will be resting on the floor; the left leg is on top of it and does not touch the floor.
3. Inhale and bring your bent knees back to the middle, placing both feet flat on the floor. Exhale and slowly lower your bent knees to the left, turning your head to the right.
4. Repeat, alternating legs, 3 times slowly. On the last repetition, hold to each side for 6 to 8 breaths. Then bring your bent knees back to the middle.

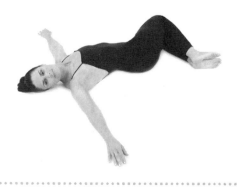

→ *Knees to Chest* ←

This posture relieves stiffness, misalignment, and discomfort in your lower back. It releases abdominal gas and relieves menstrual cramps. We are using it to compensate for the strenuous twisting of your back in the previous posture. (Note that Knees to Chest is different from Knee to Chest, which appears elsewhere in the book.)

1. Lie on your back with your knees bent, feet on the floor at hip width. Bring your bent knees toward your chest and hold on to the top of your shins, just below your knees, one hand on each knee. If you are having knee problems, hold the backs of your thighs, under your knees.
2. As you exhale, draw your knees toward your chest. As you inhale, move your knees a few inches away from your chest, rolling your hips to the floor.
3. Repeat 3 times and then stay in the folded position for 6 to 8 breaths.

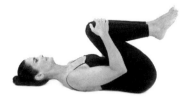

⤜ Bent-Leg Corpse with Long Exhale ⤛

This is the classic posture for relaxation of the mind–body, with bent legs to support your back.

1. Lie on your back with your arms at your sides, palms up. Bend your knees with your feet flat on the floor, approximately hip width. If you like, place pillows or rolled blankets under your knees for comfort.
2. Close your eyes and relax. If your head tilts back or your throat is tense, use a pillow or folded blanket under your head.
3. Gradually increase the length of your exhalation until you reach your comfortable maximum. Repeat for 20 to 30 breaths, and then gradually return to your resting breath for 5 to 10 breaths before you get up.

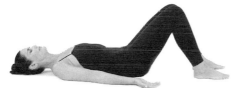

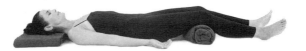

This relaxation pose promotes circulation to the legs, hips, and lower back and has a calming effect on the nervous system. You can substitute it for the Corpse if you like. You will need a chair with a sturdy level seat.

1. Lie on your back with your knees bent, feet on the floor. Place the chair (with the front edge of the seat turned toward you) just in front of your feet. Lift your feet off the floor and lay your calves on the seat, with the front edge of the seat snugged into the backs of your knees. If your head tilts back, place a blanket under your head.
2. Cover your eyes with a towel or eye bag.
3. Gradually increase the length of your exhalation until you reach your comfortable maximum. Repeat for 20 to 30 breaths, and then gradually return to your resting breath for 5 to 10 breaths before you get up.

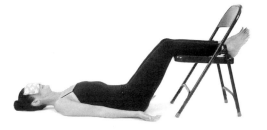

The following is a preventative program for the rehabilitation of chronic neck and upper back pain that can be used to prevent neck and back problems. When you begin, do this ten-minute routine for two to four weeks. When you are ready, add the Phase One exercises from the Lower Back Routine (page 114) for two to four weeks. The total routine should take about thirty minutes. When this is comfortable, you can use the entire Lower Back Routine instead. Use Belly Breathing (page 41) or Focused Breathing (page 39) throughout. As you become more comfortable, you can incorporate the more advanced breathing technique Victorious Breath (page 44). Ideally, practice the routine twice a day until your condition improves, then practice it once a day. When you feel your condition has subsided, you may cut down to three times a week.

Caution: This routine is not for anyone in acute or severe pain. If your pain is accompanied by other symptoms, such as numbness, tingling, or weakness in your arms, it is advisable to check with your doctor before using this program.

Seated Posture

This posture will be used for all the upper back and neck routines.

1. Sit comfortably in an armless chair, bringing your body slightly away from the back rest.
2. Let your arms hang down by your sides. Place your feet evenly on the floor at hip width. If your feet do not touch the floor, place a folded blanket or a phone book under them. Your thighs should be parallel to the floor with your knees and hips bent at approximately a 90 degree angle.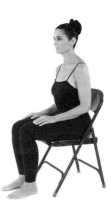
3. Place your hands on your thighs with your fingers toward your knees. Bring your back up nice and tall, and gently pull your head back until your ears, shoulders, and hip sockets are in alignment.
4. Hold for 8 to 10 breaths.

Seated Alternate Arm Raise

This simple arm movement gently stretches the muscles of the upper and lower back, working each side of the back separately, since so many back problems are asymmetrical, or one sided. It also promotes circulation to your neck and shoulders.

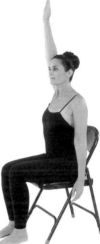

1. Start in the Seated Posture.
2. Let your arms hang at your sides, palms turned back. Look straight ahead.
3. As you inhale, raise your right arm forward and up overhead until it is vertical.
4. As you exhale, bring your right arm down to the starting position.
5. As you inhale, raise your left arm forward and up overhead. Exhale on the return.
6. Repeat 4 to 6 times, alternating arms.

Shoulder Rolls

Shoulder Rolls help increase the range of motion in your shoulder joints. Do them slowly, focusing on each part of the movement and coordinating with your breath.

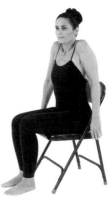

1. Start in the Seated Posture.
2. Let your arms hang at your sides, palms turned back. Look straight ahead.
3. As you inhale, roll the shoulders up and back, as if you were doing a giant shrug.
4. As you exhale, drop your shoulders down.
5. Repeat 4 to 6 times.
6. Reverse the direction and repeat 4 to 6 times.

Wing and Prayer

This simple movement gently works your upper back and opens up your chest.

1. Start in the Seated Posture.
2. As you exhale, join your palms in the prayer position, thumbs at the breast-bone.
3. As you inhale, separate your hands and stretch your arms like wings to the sides at shoulder height. Your wrists stay flexed, your fingers pointing toward the ceiling and your palms facing away from you. Look straight ahead.
4. As you exhale, join the palms again at the breastbone.
5. Repeat 4 to 6 times.

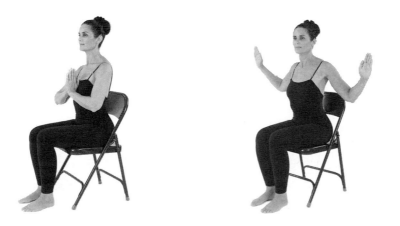

Mirror on Hand

This exercise stretches your neck and upper back.

1. Start in the Seated Posture.
2. Place your hands on your thighs, palms down. As you inhale, raise your right hand up to eye level with the fingers pointing upward and your palm facing away from you. Hold your hand at a comfortable distance, as if you were looking into a mirror on the back of your hand.
3. As you exhale, bring your right hand toward you and place the palm on the top of your left shoulder. Turn your head to the left and down, watching your hand.
4. As you inhale, move your right hand away from your shoulder at eye level, with your arm extended with your elbow slightly bent. Keep going around the front and continuing all the way to the right. Follow your hand with your eyes, and stop the movement when your head is as far as it can comfortably turn to the right.
5. As you exhale, bring your hand back in front of you as in Step 2, then lower your hand down to the starting position.
6. Repeat slowly, alternating the right and left side, 4 to 6 times each.

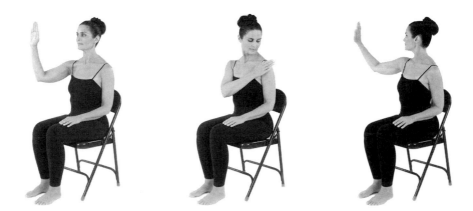

The Newspaper

This movement gently stretches your upper back and neck, while opening the chest and working the shoulders.

1. Start in the Seated Posture.
2. Place your hands on your thighs, palms up. As you exhale, raise both hands to eye level, palms facing you as though you were holding an open newspaper.
3. As you inhale, move your open hands forward, up, and overhead, keeping a slight bend in your elbows and your shoulders dropped. Follow your hands with your eyes and head. Stop when your hands are directly over your forehead.
4. As you exhale, bring only your chin down toward your chest.
5. As you inhale, bring your elbows back and apart from each other, turning your palms forward and flexing your wrists backward. Lift your chin off your chest and look straight ahead, pressing your elbows back.
6. As you exhale, round your back forward like a camel, bringing your bent arms forward so that they are in front of you. Keep a slight bend in your elbows. Your arms should be roughly parallel to the floor, with your arms and ears in alignment.
7. As you inhale, return to the starting position; then exhale.
8. Repeat 3 to 4 times.

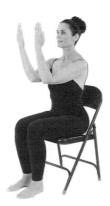 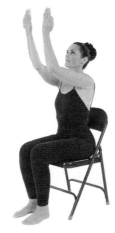

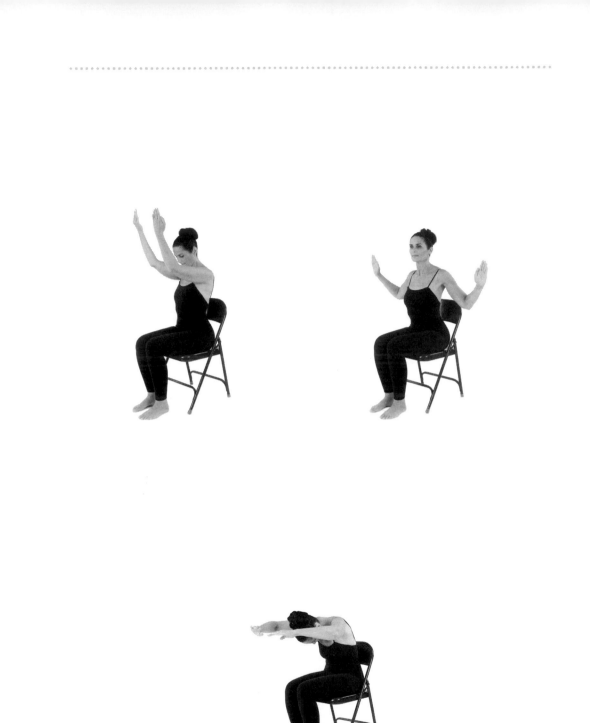

Seated Chair Twist

This gentle twisting motion promotes circulation to your back and tones the abdomen and rejuvenates the spine.

Caution: Move carefully and slowly while executing a twist. If you experience any pain or discomfort, leave the twist out of your routine until you can check with your health-care professional.

1. Sit sideways on a chair with the chair back to your right, feet flat on the floor, and heels directly below your knees.
2. Exhale, turn to the right, and hold the sides of the chair back with your hands. If your feet are not comfortably on the floor, place a folded blanket or a phone book under them.
3. As you inhale, bring your back up tall, as if you were trying to touch the ceiling with the top of your spine.
4. As you exhale, twist your torso and head farther to the right.
5. Return to the starting position. Repeat the twist, gradually twisting farther with each exhalation for 3 breaths, but do not go beyond your comfort zone. On the last repetition, hold the twist for 4 to 6 breaths; then return to the starting position.
6. Repeat the same sequence on the opposite side.

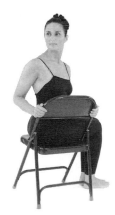

Sitting Fold

This posture stretches your lower back and flexes your hips.

1. Start in the Seated Posture.
2. As you exhale, bend forward from your hips and slide your hands forward and down your legs. Hang your head and arms down, and relax in the folded position for 6 to 8 breaths.
3. Roll your body back up to the seated position.

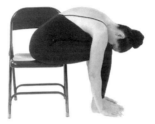

Seated Relaxation with Long Exhale

1. Start in the Seated Posture.
2. Close your eyes and begin Belly Breathing (page 41). Gradually increase the length of your exhalation until you reach your comfortable maximum.
3. Repeat for 20 to 30 breaths. Then gradually return to your normal breath for 5 to 10 breaths before you get up.

Yoga for the Knees

The following program is for the rehabilitation of injured knees. If you have had a serious injury or you are in acute pain, you should talk with your physician before practicing Yoga therapy. This routine takes approximately twenty minutes and should be practiced using Focused Breathing (page 39) or Belly Breathing (page 41). Ideally, practice the routine twice a day until your condition improves, then practice it once a day. When you feel your condition has subsided, you may cut down to three times a week.

Bent-Legs Corpse

This is the classic posture for relaxation of the body and mind, modified by bending the knees. The bent knees add support for the lower back.

1. Lie on your back with your arms at your sides, palms up. Place pillows or rolled blankets under your knees for comfort.
2. Bend your knees with your feet on the floor at hip width. If your head tilts back or if your neck or throat is tense, use a pillow or folded blanket under your head. Stay in the posture for 8 to 10 breaths.
3. Relax with your eyes closed.

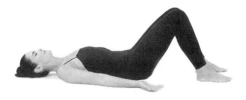

Knees to Chest (Modified)

This calming posture flexes the hips and knees and promotes circulation to your lower body.

1. Lie on your back with your knees bent, feet on the floor at hip width.
2. As you exhale, bring your bent knees toward your chest and hold on to the back of your thighs, just above your knees. You should feel a gentle stretch in your lower back and hips.
3. As you inhale, move your knees away from your chest, but do not lower them all the way to the floor.
4. Repeat 6 to 8 times, then return your legs to the floor in the bent-knee position.

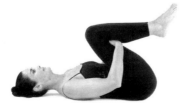

Bent-Leg Hamstring Stretch

This gentle stretch loosens up your hamstrings and flexes your hips.

1. Lie on your back with bent knees and feet on the floor at hip width. Relax your arms at your sides, palms down.
2. As you exhale, bring your right knee toward your chest, and hold the back of your right thigh with both hands just below your knee.
3. As you inhale, extend your right leg toward the ceiling as high as you feel comfortable, continuing to hold your leg. Do not force it—your knee does not need to be fully locked out. Keep your foot flexed.
4. As you exhale, return your leg to the bent position. Keep your head and the top of your hips on the floor. Place a pillow or blanket under your head if the back of your head tilts back or your throat tenses while raising or lowering the leg.
5. Repeat the leg extension 3 to 4 times. Then hold your extended leg with your hands interlaced on the back of the thigh for 6 to 8 breaths.
6. Lower your right foot to the floor.
7. Repeat with the left leg.

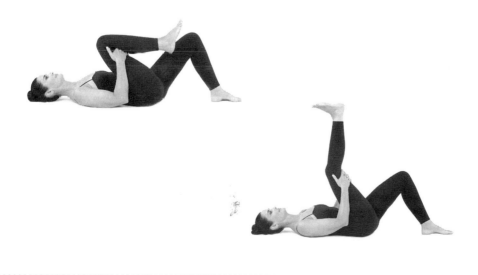

Yoga Crunches

This exercise strengthens and tones your abdomen, especially the upper part above the navel. It also strengthens the inside of your thighs (adductors) as well as your neck and shoulders.

1. Lie on your back, bend your knees, and place your feet on the floor at hip width.
2. Turn your heels out and toes in (pigeon-toed). Tilt your inner knees together until they touch.
3. Interlace your fingers behind your head, and hook your thumbs under the angle of the jawbone, slightly below the ears.
4. As you exhale, push your knees together firmly, tilt your pelvis toward your navel, and use your abdominal muscles to slowly sit up, keeping your hips on the floor. Go only halfway up, so that about half your back is off the floor. Keep your elbows wide and to the sides, in alignment with the tops of your shoulders, using your hands to support your head. Look toward the tops of your knees. Do not pull your head up with your arms.
5. As you inhale, slowly roll back down.
6. Repeat 6 to 8 times.

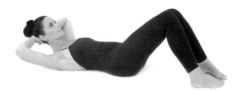

Reclined Bound Angle

This simple exercise stretches and tones the insides of your thighs (adductors) and groin. It also helps bring circulation to the pelvis area and the lower back.

1. Lie on your back with your knees bent, feet flat on the floor 8 to 12 inches from your buttocks. Place your hands at your sides, palms down.
2. As you inhale, slowly open your legs wide toward the floor, and join the soles of your feet together. You should feel a nice gentle stretch in your inner thighs.
3. As you exhale, slowly bring your knees back together.
4. Repeat 3 times, then stay in the open position (Step 2) for 6 to 8 breaths. Then bring your knees back together.

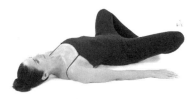

Seated Leg Raise

This seated posture strengthens your thighs, the deep hip flexors (psoas), and the muscles of the legs that support your knees.

1. Sit on the floor with your legs extended in front of you and with your back up tall. Place a tightly rolled Yoga mat or folded blanket under your knees. Put your palms on the floor behind you with your fingers pointing toward your hips, or put your back up against a wall.

2. As you exhale, tighten your right thigh and flex your right foot. Point your toes back toward you, extending your right heel forward as if you were pushing against something solid. Hold for 5 to 8 seconds, continuing to exhale.

3. Inhale. Then slowly exhale, keeping your right leg firm and raising it until the right heel is just above the toes of the left foot. Hold for another 5 to 8 seconds, continuing to exhale. Don't force it, just raise your leg as high as possible. Keep your chest lifted and your shoulders dropped.

4. As you inhale, relax your right leg and bring it back down to the starting position.

5. Repeat with the left leg, and then alternate 6 to 8 times on each leg.

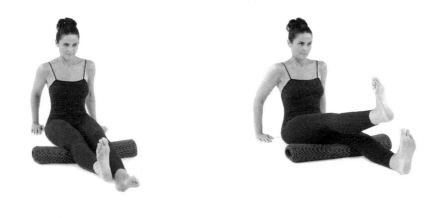

Locust with Support (Modified)

The posture strengthens your hamstrings and the muscles that support the back of your knee and your buttocks. It is a nice stretch for your lower back.

1. Lie on your belly, with a folded blanket under your hips and rib cage to prevent hyperextending your lower back. Keep your legs slightly apart with the tops of your feet on the floor.
2. Place your forearms on the floor in front of you, parallel with each other, with your elbows aligned below your shoulders.
3. As you inhale, raise your chest to a comfortable level supported by your forearms, and then raise your right leg backward as high as comfortable.
4. As you exhale, bend the right leg, bringing your heel toward the buttocks, until your leg makes a right angle.
5. As you inhale, straighten the right leg. Repeat Steps 4 and 5, for 6 to 8 times. Rest for a few moments on your belly as in Step 1; then repeat the entire sequence with the left leg.

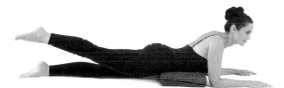

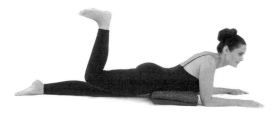

Knees to Chest (Modified)

This posture is repeated in this routine to increase circulation to the hips and knees. It should feel great in your lower back.

1. Lie on your back with your knees bent, feet on the floor at hip width.
2. As you exhale, bring your bent knees toward your chest and hold on to the back of your thighs, just above your knees. You should feel a gentle stretch in your lower back and hips.
3. As you inhale, move your knees away from your chest, but do not lower them all the way to the floor.
4. Repeat 6 to 8 times, then return your legs to the floor in the bent-knee position.

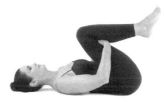

Legs on a Chair

This relaxation technique uses a chair to improve circulation to your feet, legs, hips, and lower back. It has a calming effect on your nervous system.

1. Place a chair in an area where you have room to lie down in front of it.
2. Lie on your back with your knees bent, feet on the floor. The front edge of the chair's seat should be turned toward you, just in front of your feet.
3. Lift your feet off the floor, and lay your calves on the chair seat, with the front edge of the seat tucked into the backs of your knees. If your head tilts back, place a blanket under it.
4. Use Belly Breathing (page 41) with a long exhale or the Healing Triangles (page 52) for 20 to 30 breaths.

Yoga for Arthritis

The following program helps manage the pain of arthritis. This routine is designed to increase circulation and range of motion in your joints. If you have arthritis in your knees or back, use the specific routines for those body parts, given earlier in this chapter. For arthritis of the hands, arms, and feet, use this routine. The program takes approximately twenty minutes and should be practiced using Focused Breathing (page 39). Ideally, practice the routine twice a day until your condition improves, then practice it once a day. When you feel your condition has subsided, you may cut down to three times a week.

. . . .

Seated Posture

This simple seated posture helps relax your nervous system and link your body, breath, and mind in preparation for the subsequent exercises. You will be using this posture for much of this routine.

1. Sit comfortably in a sturdy armless chair, bringing your body slightly away from the back rest.
2. Let your arms hang down by your sides. Place your feet evenly on the floor at hip width. If your feet do not touch the floor, place a folded blanket or a phone book under them. Your thighs should be parallel to the floor with your knees and hips bent at approximately a 90 degree angle.
3. Place your hands on your thighs with your fingers toward your knees. Draw your head slightly back, centering it over your shoulders and your torso. Imagine a straight line running vertically from your ears, straight down through your shoulders and ending at your hips. Keep this line straight, but don't force yourself into any position that's uncomfortable.
4. Use Focused Breathing for 8 to 10 breaths.

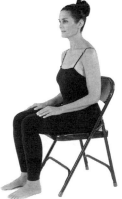

. . . .

Seated Alternate Arm Raise

This simple exercise can be energizing while improving the range of motion in your shoulder joints.

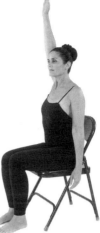

1. Start in the Seated Posture.
2. Let your arms hang at your sides, palms turned back. Look straight ahead.
3. As you inhale, raise your right arm forward and up overhead until it is vertical.
4. As you exhale, bring your right arm down to the starting position.
5. As you inhale, raise your left arm forward and up overhead. Exhale on the return.
6. Repeat 6 to 8 times, alternating arms.

Shoulder Rolls

Shoulder Rolls are often used in exercise programs, because they help the range of motion in the shoulder joints. Here we do them slowly, focusing on each part of the movement and coordinating it with the breath.

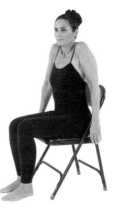

1. Start in the Seated Posture.
2. Let your arms hang at your sides, palms turned back. Look straight ahead.
3. As you inhale, roll the shoulders up and back, as if you were doing a giant shrug.
4. As you exhale, drop your shoulders down.
5. Repeat 4 to 6 times.
6. Reverse the direction and repeat 4 to 6 times.

Hand Clenching

This exercise increases blood flow and improves range of motion in your hand, wrist, and finger joints.

1. Start in the Seated Posture.
2. Keeping your right arm straight, bring it up and out in front of you to the height of your shoulder, parallel to the floor. Make a fist with the thumb side up, and tuck your thumb down into the fingers.
3. As you inhale, open the hand, and then stretch all five fingers as if you were trying to touch all the walls in the room at one time.
4. As you exhale, fold the hand back up, with the thumb tucked in.
5. Repeat 6 to 8 times.
6. Repeat with the left hand.
7. Do two rounds with each hand. After you are familiar with the sequence, use both hands at the same time for two rounds.

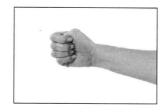 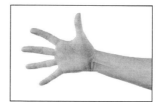

Wrist Bending

This simple exercise improves the range of motion of the wrist.

1. Start in the Seated Posture.
2. Bring your right arm and hand up in front of you to the height of your shoulder, parallel to the floor. Turn the palm of your right hand down and extend your fingers and thumb forward and close together.
3. As you inhale, bend your right hand at the wrist backward as though you were pressing your hand against a wall.
4. As you exhale, bend your hand down at the wrist to your comfortable maximum. You should feel a light pull all the way up your forearm.
5. Repeat 6 to 8 times.
6. Repeat with the left hand.
7. Do two rounds with each hand. When you are familiar with the sequence, use both hands at the same time for two rounds.

Wrist-Joint Rotation

This rotation exercise improves the range of motion of your wrist.

1. Start in the Seated Posture.
2. Bring your right arm and hand up in front of you to the height of your shoulder, parallel to the floor. Make a fist, with your thumb tucked into the fingers and your palm down.
3. Let your breath be free and begin to rotate your right wrist in clockwise circles 6 to 8 times, keeping your arm motionless.
4. Change directions and rotate your wrist counterclockwise 6 to 8 times.
5. Repeat the sequence with the left hand.
6. Do two rounds with each hand. When you are comfortable with the sequence, work both wrists at the same time for two rounds.

Seated Ankle Bending

This exercise loosens up the ankles and feet, improving circulation and flexibility.

1. Sit on the floor comfortably with your legs extended in front of you. Place the palms of your hands on the floor behind you with the fingers pointing toward your hips or lean your back against a wall.
2. Flex your right foot back toward you so it sticks up at a right angle to the floor.
3. As you exhale, point your right foot and toes forward and down.
4. As you inhale, bring your foot back to the right-angle position.
5. Repeat 8 to 10 times for two rounds.
6. Repeat with the left foot. When you are comfortable with the routine, do both feet at the same time for two rounds.

Seated Ankle Rotation

Rotating the ankle increases its flexibility and blood flow.

1. Sit on the floor with your legs extended in front of you. Place a tightly rolled Yoga mat or folded blanket under your knees. Put the palms of your hands on the floor behind you with your fingers pointing toward your hips, or lean your back against a wall.
2. Flex your right foot back toward you at a right angle with the floor.
3. Let your breath be free and slowly rotate your foot clockwise at the ankle joint 8 to 10 times. Reverse it and rotate counterclockwise 8 to 10 times. Do two sets each, then repeat with the left foot for two sets.
4. When you are comfortable with the routine, do both feet at the same time for two sets.

Legs on a Chair

This relaxation technique calms the nervous system, while increasing blood flow to the feet, legs, hips, and lower back. You will need a chair with a sturdy level seat.

1. Place a chair in an area where you have room to lie down in front of it.
2. Lie on your back with your knees bent, feet on the floor. The front edge of chair's seat should be turned toward you, just in front of your feet.
3. Lift your feet off the floor, and lay your calves on the chair seat, with the front edge of the seat tucked into the backs of your knees. If your head tilts back, place a blanket under it.
4. Use Belly Breathing (page 41) with a long exhale for 20 to 30 breaths.

8

The Respiratory System: Allergies, Asthma,
Bronchitis, the Common Cold

I n the Yoga tradition, breath equals life. As long as a person is breathing, they are said to be alive. The body's breathing center is known as the respiratory system, and its health is a major focus of all Yoga practice.

But what happens when something goes wrong with your respiratory system? Fortunately, not only can you continue to practice Yoga but you can use Yoga therapy to manage and sometimes heal your respiratory problems.

Leslie is a forty-nine-year-old Yoga teacher and registered nurse who grew up in Boston but now lives in Los Angeles. From the age of three, she has been plagued by respiratory problems ignited by allergic reactions. At five she was admitted to the hospital for her first episode of "bronchitis." As a teenager, her symptoms increased when she began smoking cigarettes and her family adopted a cat. As a college student, she was diagnosed with multiple allergies and asthma, after which she began to receive allergy shots and started taking prescription medications. Over the next few years she made several visits to the emergency room for difficulty breathing.

In her late twenties and early thirties, Leslie finally gave up smoking, began to practice Yoga, improved her diet, and moved from Boston to Los Angeles for the warmer climate. With these changes she experienced significant relief from her symptoms, although she still had occasional allergic reactions. For two years she was able to eliminate her regular medication and use only alternative treatments, including Yoga and homeopathy, but when her symptoms returned she restarted medications. Leslie then began a more advanced program of Yoga therapy and fine-tuned her diet, discovering that a diet that included animal protein and was high in veggies and whole grains made a big difference in her breathing.

"Today I practice Yoga and meditation five or six days a week, combined with moderate aerobic exercises," Leslie explains. "I've found some herbs that seem to help, and I eat a healthy diet. I still take traditional medication and occasional allergy shots, but my respiratory flare-ups are far less frequent, and my quality of life is better than it has ever been." Leslie illustrates perfectly the Yoga philosophy of taking the holistic approach to healing. Through experimentation and remaining open to different ideas, she has found a recipe that combines Yoga, diet, and medication to effectively manage her serious asthma and allergies.

ANATOMY 101

The Respiratory System

The respiratory system consists of the nose, mouth, sinuses, and lungs, plus the various air passages (including the larynx, trachea, and bronchi). Its main purpose is to take in air, extract oxygen, and get rid of carbon dioxide. The respiratory system is also what allows you to speak.

Your nose serves the important function of warming, moisturizing, and filtering the air. The mucous membranes of the nose have a good blood supply to keep them warm and capable of producing a moist mucous lining. The visible hairs and the small invisible hairs (called cilia) act as filters to keep dirt and particles out of your intake system, kind of like the air filter in a car.

The sinuses are air spaces that are lined with the same mucous membranes as the nose. Unfortunately, these air spaces are prone to infection and tend to cause problems during allergies and respiratory illnesses, such as when you get a cold.

The mouth is shared by the respiratory system and the digestive system. When your nose is blocked, you breathe through your mouth, a nice backup system for your body's most crucial function. "The nose is meant for breathing and the mouth is meant for eating" is a Yoga axiom that makes sense, because the nose delivers higher-quality air to the lungs. It's important that the air you breathe is warm, moist, and clean; conversely, cool, dry, or dirty air can be a cause of respiratory problems. So it's best to inhale through the nose when you can.

The larynx is also called your voice box because it contains the vocal cords. Speech and vocal sounds are created when air leaving the lungs passes over the vocal cords, causing them to vibrate. It is the vibration of these vocal cords that allows us to speak, sing, and chant. When the vocal cords are in use, they narrow the air passage and can slow the release of air from the lungs. This is one of the reasons chanting is common in Yoga—to produce a long, slow exhalation of breath.

The trachea is a large air tube that leads from the larynx to the lungs. The bronchi are the smaller air passages that lead from the trachea to the many parts of the lungs. They branch into the smaller bronchioles, which ultimately lead to the lung tissue. The bronchi look like the branches of an upside-down tree. These air passages can become irritated by infections, allergies, and asthma. The irritation or inflammation can lead to narrowing of these passages, making it hard to move air into and out of the lung.

Everyone's respiratory system gets compromised at one time or another. The most common problems are allergies, asthma, bronchitis, and the common cold. Note that both medical and Yoga practitioners emphasize the importance of an overall healthy lifestyle to prevent and manage respiratory illness. A good diet, exercise, and avoidance of smoking can go a long way toward avoiding all of the common respiratory problems. Yoga is an effective addition to such a healthy lifestyle.

RESPIRATORY AILMENTS

Allergies

If you're subject to frequent allergy attacks, your immune system operates on over-drive—following a set of faulty instructions. When a substance that is normally harmless causes your immune system to react as if the substance were harmful, you have an allergic reaction. The body goes on attack to expel the substance and protect itself from danger. Anything that causes this dysfunctional immune response is called an allergen.

The tendency to be allergic is hereditary, though specific allergies are not. If you have an allergy, there's a good chance that at least one of your parents is also allergic to something. Allergies affect more than 20 percent of the U.S. population, making them the sixth leading cause of chronic illness.[1]

It is common for allergy sufferers to report that their symptoms worsen when they're under unusual stress. For some people, any heightened negative emotion such as anger or depression can intensify their allergies. This is a key to understanding why the stress-relieving effects of Yoga can be a tremendous advantage for allergy sufferers.

Because allergies have no single cause or precipitating factor and the triggers vary so much with the individual, the Yoga perspective is that allergies must be controlled by the individual who is suffering from them—as opposed to a physician, Yoga therapist, or any other health practitioner. This is true for asthma as well. You should definitely be under a doctor's care, and Yoga therapy can be a big help in managing allergies and asthma. But only *you* can control whether or not you practice Yoga and other recommended exercises, only *you* can control your food intake and avoid your triggers, and only *you* can control your exposure to detrimental environmental factors (pollution, tobacco smoke, pollen, dust). If you suffer from allergies, be sure to read The Yoga Prescription for Respiratory Ailments on page 160 and Yoga for Allergies on page 162.

Asthma

Recent Centers for Disease Control and Prevention (CDC) reports indicate that at least fifteen million American adults have asthma, including about 10 percent of the athletes who competed in the 1996 Olympics. Numerous big stars in professional football, baseball, and basketball have asthma, and track star Jackie Joyner-Kersee has written about her asthma in publications including the *New York Times*.[2] The one thing all these asthma sufferers have in common is that to preserve their quality of life, they actively manage their disease through medical supervision and various self-help techniques including exercise, diet, and stress control, and they don't smoke.

Asthma is a constriction of the air passages within the lungs. Airways become inflamed and then go on to become narrowed. It is the narrow airways that cause the wheezing sound and make it difficult to breathe. The constriction is reversible—it can come and go. When you are having an asthma attack, you may feel like your lungs are burning, something heavy is crushing your chest, or something is choking your neck. You may cough, gasp, or wheeze all in the effort to breathe.

Yoga can be particularly helpful for asthma sufferers since it centers on deep, focused breathing and tension relief, which can help people deal with the fear factor of asthma by providing calming strategies to enhance airflow. Relaxation techniques can also help counter the anxiety that might accompany an asthma attack. Yoga breathing can help you feel more in control, both between and during asthma attacks. It is important to note that during an asthma attack, modern medicine is the best treatment.

As mentioned in the discussion of allergies, ancient Yoga wisdom places you, the asthma sufferer, at the center of responsibility for your own healing. Your case of asthma is unique, your triggers and symptoms highly individual, so you will find you can manage your attacks and symptoms if you take the holistic view—integrating conventional medications with attention to diet, exercise, and your environment. As is true with allergies, you are in a better position than anyone else to keep your asthma under control. If you suffer from asthma, be sure to read The Yoga Prescription for Respiratory Ailments on page 160, and Yoga for Asthma and Bronchitis on page 162.

Bronchitis

You've had a cold for more than ten days, and now you have a fever and a nasty cough yielding some wonderfully colored phlegm. You finally go see the doctor and get the diagnosis: bronchitis. Usually beginning with an upper respiratory virus (a cold), bronchitis is the inflammation of the bronchial tree. The infection leads to a phlegm-producing cough and sometimes narrowed airways. Bronchitis can be viral or bacterial.

Acute bronchitis usually clears up on its own within five to seven days, but many doctors will prescribe antibiotics just in case there is a bacterial infection. If the symptoms linger longer than a couple of weeks or occur for three months out of the year, two years in a row, the diagnosis is chronic bronchitis. If you tend to get bronchitis following colds, be sure to read The Yoga Prescription for Respiratory Ailments on page 160 and Yoga for Asthma and Bronchitis on page 162.

The Common Cold

The common cold is a respiratory infection principally affecting the nose. It is caused by a virus, meaning that antibiotics don't help it. Researchers estimate there may be over a hundred rhinoviruses and other respiratory viruses that cause colds.

Colds strike American adults an average of two or three times a year with symptoms lasting four or five days. Young children get colds four to eight times a year and often hang on to their symptoms for more than a week. Parents of young children get more colds than other adults, and people over the age of sixty usually get less than one cold a year, probably because of their built-up immunity and lack of exposure to as many viruses.

Contrary to what your grandmother may have told you, you can't catch a cold from being out in cold weather. "Cold season" probably occurs in the winter months because of the extra time spent indoors in closer contact with other people, giving the virus more opportunity to spread. Cold weather also dries the air, helping the cold virus to thrive and at the same time making your nasal passages more susceptible to infection. Colds are most often transmitted through the hands—by touching something or someone who carries the virus and then touching your eyes, nose, or mouth. You can also catch a cold by inhaling the airborne particles ejected by somebody when they cough or sneeze. However, the strength of your immune system is one of the most important determinants of whether or not you will catch a cold.

Ancient Yoga wisdom views the common cold as your body's natural way of eliminating impurities. It is true that the symptoms of a cold—increased mucus production, coughing, and sneezing—are your respiratory system's efforts to cleanse itself of the cold virus. While there are many things we can do to strengthen the immune system and increase the body's effectiveness at resisting and fighting colds, the only sure-fire cure is the passage of time. If you suffer from frequent colds, be sure to read The Yoga Prescription for Respiratory Ailments on page 160 and Yoga for the Common Cold on page 171.

The Yoga Advantage for Respiratory Ailments

Joe is a semiretired businessman in his early sixties who first showed up in my group class wearing a Harley-Davidson T-shirt. He was heavily muscled and tried too hard in all the postures. His mind-set was similar to many ex-jock macho men at their first Yoga class. I can relate to this kind of guy, so I introduced myself and told him about my own first class and how I felt out of place. He explained that his wife had been taking my class and convinced him to come because he was so stiff from weightlifting. Joe showed up twice a week like clockwork. I began to notice his improvement after about a month, and by three months he had made significant progress in all of the postures.

After attending my class for six months, he came up to me after class and told me that he had suffered from constant allergy attacks for twelve years. But after his third month of practicing Yoga, the attacks had completely vanished. He had waited three months to tell me, he said, "Because I couldn't believe it and wanted to be sure it wasn't just a fluke." I had long been aware of Yoga's rehabilitating effects on respiratory problems and was very happy it had worked so well for his allergies.

For centuries, holistic practitioners have successfully used Yoga to control respiratory ailments. Since the 1990s, medical research has verified Yoga's effectiveness in a number of studies. Research has shown that a fifteen-week program of

Yoga—including postures, breathing techniques, and relaxation—significantly improved the functioning of the lungs.[3] A number of other studies involving people with asthma have indicated that even a brief Yoga program can result in better exercise tolerance, better heart and lung function, and considerably less use of inhalers and other medication. The research has also shown across-the-board improvement in general relaxation and positive attitude after several weeks of regular Yoga practice, as reported by individuals involved in the studies.[4]

In addition to revealing scientifically that Yoga really helps people with respiratory ailments, doctors have been able to pinpoint a number of reasons it works. One of the ways in which we measure the function of the lung is to test the flow rate of air going in and out of the lung. With asthma, the flow rates are decreased, which is one of the reasons sufferers feel short of breath during an attack. Practicing Yoga has been shown to increase people's flow rates, not only during the exercise session but all the time.[5]

Respiratory disorders can also decrease vital capacity, which is a measure of the amount of air you can inhale after trying to expel all the air out of your lungs. A regular practice of Yoga increases your vital capacity, helping you exchange air more efficiently and, in the case of asthma or bronchitis, feel less short of breath.[6]

One of the major reasons Yoga can be so effective for respiratory ailments is the stress factor. Allergies, asthma, and colds all strike more viciously when you are under stress, and Yoga is well known as a general stress reliever. When used regularly, especially with breathing and relaxation techniques, Yoga can reduce your stress enough to make an appreciable difference in your respiratory health.

There is plenty of research showing that regular exercise strengthens the heart and lungs. For people with asthma and chronic bronchitis, doctors recommend short but frequent exercise sessions to help improve breathing. Regular physical activity can decrease the frequency and severity of asthma attacks, reduce the use of medications, and improve your quality of life. In fact, while allergy and asthma sufferers are cautioned to avoid their triggers as much as possible, they are at the same time told *not* to avoid physical activity.

The exercise, relaxation, and stress reduction that naturally result from Yoga also give a big boost to your immune system. Studies have established that exercise reinforces the immune system by increasing the number and strength of immune cells and slowing the release of stress hormones. The strength of your immune system is one of the most important determinants of whether you will catch a cold, and it also affects your susceptibility to allergies and asthma attacks. Most people who regularly practice Yoga report that they get fewer colds.

Perhaps the biggest reason Yoga is so therapeutic for respiratory problems is that it involves so much more than just doing a series of postures. The lifestyle changes that naturally accompany a Yoga program can work together to bring about positive health results. I had a forty-one-year-old client named Mia who had enjoyed good health until two years before seeing me. Her thirteen-year-old son, Dominic, had switched from a small school to a large public school and began to have frequent colds, which he passed on to his mother. In talking with them, it became clear that their diet was high in fat, including many fast foods and sweets. In addition, neither of them got enough sleep, particularly when they had bad colds. Mia always tried to power through with over the counter remedies, never slowing down to give her body the extra rest it needed. This led to serious chest infections, frequent trips to her doctor, and rounds of antibiotics. Her immune system was shot, and she had little energy for social activities.

We started by cleaning up Mia and Dominic's diet, and they both agreed to earlier bedtimes. They began practicing the Core Routines (Chapter 6) to build stamina and fortify their immune systems. I also gave Mia a separate Breathing Break (described later in this chapter) to strengthen her chest and lungs. After two months, they began attending my group Yoga class twice a week, while continuing their daily practice at home. The results were truly heartwarming. Mia went the next eleven months without a cold, and Dominic lasted nine months. In the following year, Dominic had one cold and his mother had none. By embracing the holistic Yoga philosophy and applying it wherever it fit their lives, they made meaningful improvements in their health and learned what an impact a few significant changes can make.

As long as there are allergens, tobacco smoke, pollutants, and viruses lurking in our environment, most of us will never be completely free of colds, allergies, or other respiratory problems. But Yoga therapy in the context of an overall holistic health program can greatly increase our resistance to such problems and help us manage them when they do occur.

✳ Do aerobic exercise in addition to Yoga. If you are out of shape, start slowly, working up to a thirty-minute session, three to five days a week. Find types of exercise that you enjoy to increase your likelihood of following through.

✳ When you have a cold, exercise *moderately* and continue to practice your Yoga routine, if you feel able and you don't have a fever or flu symptoms.

✳ Drink lots of liquids to stay well hydrated, which will keep airway secretions thinner and easier to expel.

✳ To help keep your immune system strong, eat a diet rich in fresh fruits, vegetables, and whole grains, and try to avoid foods high in saturated fats. If you like, you can include plenty of garlic, which many people believe acts as a mild natural antibiotic.

✳ Listen to Grandma—she knew best! Certain foods can shorten the duration of symptoms associated with the common cold. Hot liquids such as tea or lemon water warm and moisten your respiratory system, thereby calming symptoms. There is even a study that indicates that chicken soup helps colds resolve more quickly.[7]

✳ Get plenty of sleep, and remember that your body needs extra rest when you are ill.

✳ Try to avoid viruses by washing your hands frequently, especially when people around you have colds.

✳ Practice the appropriate Yoga therapy routine from this chapter or from Chapter 6. Start with two or three days a week, working toward five to six days a week.

For Asthma or Allergies

✳ Learn to recognize the conditions, foods, allergens, drugs, and emotional situations that trigger allergies or asthma attacks for you, and strategize how to avoid them.

✳ Swim or do water aerobics because the water tends to moisten the air. Dry air usually makes asthma worse.

✳ Try sports that involve brief intervals of activity with rests in between—racquet sports, volleyball, softball, and golf, for example.

✳ Walking is a great aerobic exercise. Running can be problematic if it is too vigorous and doesn't incorporate periods of rest. (However, many athletes have succeeded despite respiratory problems by working with their physician to manage their condition, often taking medication before exercise.)

YOGA FOR RESPIRATORY AILMENTS

Yoga for Allergies

Once per day, practice Core Routine I (page 62). When you feel ready, switch o Core Routine II (page 78). For the relaxation at the end of the routine, practice the Healing Triangles (page 52).

Breathing Break

Once per day, practice the Shining Skull Breath (page 46) or Alternate Nostril Breathing (page 45) for three to ten minutes.

Yoga for Asthma and Bronchitis

This routine is similar to the one I first gave Leslie (page 151), who suffered from serious asthma and allergies. It is less strenuous than the Core Routines described in Chapter 6. The breathing and the folding postures help people with asthma learn to push their air out effectively. This routine takes approximately fifteen minutes and should be practiced using Belly Breathing (page 41). When you feel comfortable with this routine, you can graduate to the Core Routines. Ideally, practice the routine twice a day until your condition improves, then practice it once a day. When you feel your condition has subsided, you may cut down to three times a week.

Note: This routine is not for acute conditions of asthma or bronchitis.

Seated Posture

Use this posture whenever a seated position is indicated in this routine.

1. Sit comfortably in an armless chair, bringing your body slightly away from the back rest.

2. Let your arms hang down by your sides. Place your feet evenly on the floor at hip width. If your feet do not touch the floor, place a folded blanket or a phone book under them. Your thighs should be parallel to the floor, with your knees and hips bent at approximately a 90 degree angle.

3. Place your hands on your thighs with your fingers toward your knees. Bring your back up nice and tall, and gently pull your head back until your ears, shoulders, and hip sockets are in alignment. Do not force anything beyond your comfort level.

4. Use Belly Breathing (page 41) for 8 to 10 breaths. Gently draw the belly in on the exhale.

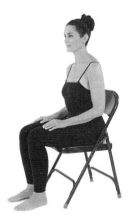

Seated Alternate Arm Raise

This simple exercise can be energizing while it improves the range of motion in your shoulder joints.

1. Start in the Seated Posture.
2. Let your arms hang at your sides, palms turned back. Look straight ahead.
3. As you inhale, raise your right arm forward and up overhead until it is vertical.
4. As you exhale, bring your right arm down to the starting position.
5. As you inhale, raise your left arm forward and up overhead. Exhale on the return.
6. Repeat 4 to 6 times, alternating arms.

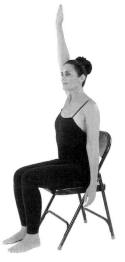

Wing and Prayer (Extended)

This movement gently works the upper back and opens up the chest.

1. Start in the Seated Posture.
2. As you exhale, join your palms in the prayer position, thumbs at your breast-bone.
3. As you inhale, raise your joined hands overhead. Follow your thumbs with your eyes.
4. As you exhale, bring your hands back to your breastbone, as in Step 2.
5. As you inhale, separate your hands and stretch your arms like wings to the sides at shoulder height. Look straight ahead.
6. As you exhale, join your palms again at the breastbone.
7. Repeat the entire sequence 4 to 6 times.

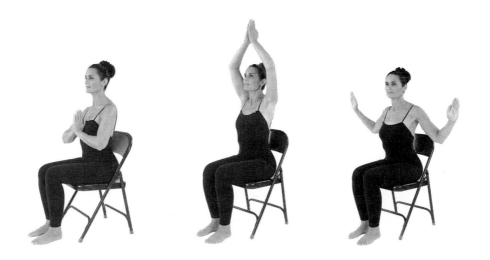

The Newspaper

This movement stretches the upper back and neck, while opening the chest and working the shoulders.

1. Start in the Seated Posture, with your palms up.
2. Place your hands on your thighs, palms up. As you exhale, raise both hands to eye level, palms facing you as though you were holding an open newspaper.
3. As you inhale, move your open hands forward, up, and overhead. Follow your hands with your eyes and head. Stop when your hands are directly over your forehead.
4. As you exhale, bring only your chin down toward your chest.
5. As you inhale, bring your elbows back and apart from each other, turning your palms forward and flexing your wrists backward. Lift your chin off your chest and look straight ahead, pressing your elbows back.
6. As you exhale, round your back forward like a camel, bringing your bent arms forward so that they are in front of you. Keep a slight bend in your elbows. Your arms should be roughly parallel with the floor, with your arms and ears in alignment.
7. As you inhale, return to the starting position; then fully exhale.
8. Repeat 4 to 6 times.

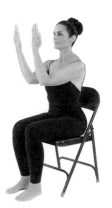
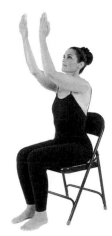

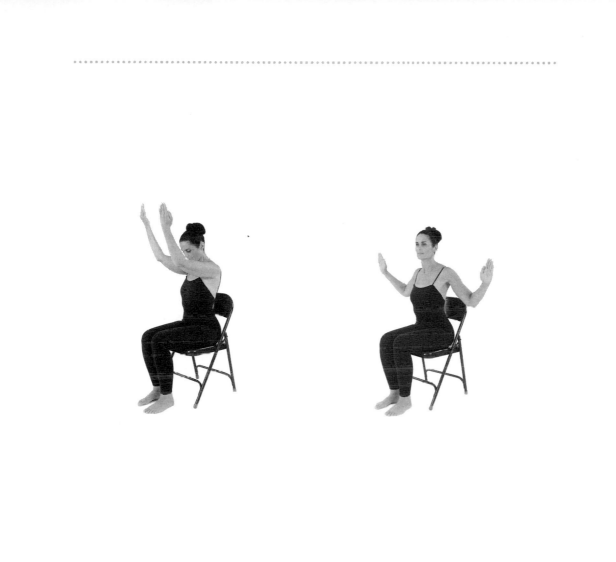

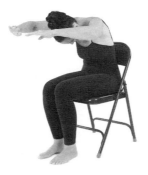

Seated Chair Twist

This gentle twisting motion promotes circulation in your back, tones your abdomen, and refreshes your lungs.

1. Sit sideways on a chair with the chair back to your right, feet flat on the floor, and heels directly below your knees.
2. Exhale, turn to the right, and grasp the sides of the chair back with your hands. If your feet are not comfortably on the floor, place a folded blanket or a phone book under them.
3. As you inhale, bring your back up tall, as if you were trying to touch the ceiling with the top of your spine.
4. As you exhale, twist your torso and head farther to the right.
5. Return to the starting position. Repeat the twist, gradually twisting farther with each exhalation for 3 breaths, but do not go beyond your comfort zone. On the last repetition, hold the twist for 4 to 6 breaths; then return to the starting position.
6. Repeat the same sequence on the opposite side.

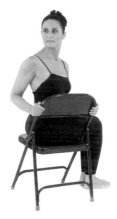

Sitting Fold

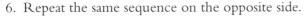

This posture stretches your lower back and helps expel air from the lungs effectively.

1. Start in the Seated Posture.
2. As you exhale, bend forward from your hips and slide your hands forward and down your legs. Let your head and arms hang down, and relax in the folded position.
3. Slowly come up and repeat 3 times. Then stay in the folded position for 6 to 8 breaths. Slowly come up.

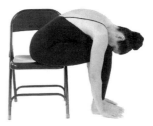

Two-Step Exhalation

This exercise is good for strengthening your lungs and gaining control of your breathing.

1. Start in the Seated Posture.
2. Inhale fully; then exhale half of your breath in 3 to 5 seconds.
3. Hold your breath for 3 to 5 seconds.
4. Exhale the remaining breath as you draw your belly inward.
5. Repeat 8 to 10 times.

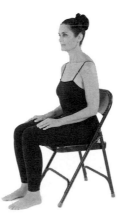

Legs on a Chair with Solar Visualization

This posture is for relaxation and helps you transition out of your Yoga routine.

1. Place a chair in an area where you have room to lie down in front of it.
2. Lie on your back with your knees bent, feet on the floor. The front edge of the chair's seat should be turned toward you, just in front of your feet.
3. Lift your feet off the floor, and lay your calves on the chair seat, with the front edge of the seat tucked into the back of your knees. If your head tilts back, place a blanket under it. Cover your eyes with a towel or eye bag.
4. As you inhale, visualize the healing rays of the sun warming and healing your chest and lungs. As you exhale, visualize darkness, impurities, and ill-health leaving your body.
5. Repeat for 3 to 5 minutes, and then slowly bring your focus back to the moment. Bend your knees toward your body, taking your legs off the chair. Roll to one side, and then onto your hands and knees. Wait 1 to 2 minutes before you stand up.

Breathing Break

Once per day, practice Two-Step Exhalation (page 169) for three to ten minutes.

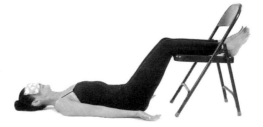

Yoga for the Common Cold

Practice Core Routine II (page 78) once daily, five to seven days a week, to build up the immune system and increase stamina. At the end of the routine, use the Healing Triangles (page 52) for your relaxation technique. If Core Routine II is too difficult, practice Core Routine I or the easier Lower Back Routine (page 114) for about two to four weeks each, and work up to Core Routine II.

Breathing Break

Once per day, practice the Shining Skull Breath (page 46) and Alternate Nostril Breathing (page 45), for three to five minutes each.

When you are in the acute stage of a cold, it is important that your body receives the proper rest so that it can heal itself. Practice the Corpse two or three times a day when you have a cold.

The Corpse

This is the classic posture for deep rest.

1. Lie flat on your back with your arms relaxed near your sides and palms turned up. Close your eyes and relax. If your head tilts back or your neck is uncomfortable, place a small pillow or blanket under your head and neck. If your lower back is uncomfortable, place a pillow or rolled blanket under your knees.
2. Use the Yoga Nidra (page 53) relaxation technique for 5 to 20 minutes.

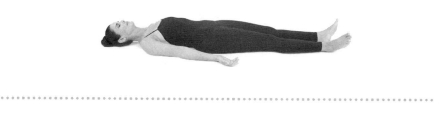

9

The Circulatory System:

High Blood Pressure, Heart Disease

Chuck Rosin is a television executive, known in the industry for his talent as a writer and producer. By his early forties he had helped create some of Hollywood's most popular television series, but along the way he suffered a heart attack and after an angioplasty procedure, another artery closure. It was a big wake-up call, and with a little nudging from his wife, Karen, and the support of his cardiologist, he decided it was time to make some changes and try Yoga. I will never forget his responses to the questionnaire we gave him. Under the question "Why have you come to the Samata Yoga Center?" he wrote, "Prevent death for as long as possible."

I think it is fair to say that in the beginning, Yoga was not Chuck's thing. He was extremely tense and reluctant to slow himself down. We started with some very simple relaxation techniques in the Corpse posture, a serene but very effective posture described in this chapter. Chuck also began making small changes in his lifestyle as he felt ready for them. Because he had a high cholesterol level, he reduced the fat in his diet. His cardiologist also prescribed a medication to lower his cholesterol. He exercised on the treadmill three times a week, and on sunny days he swam. After a few weeks, he graduated to the Lower Back Routine (page 114) and then after another month we included the Neck and Upper Back Routine (page 129) as well, which he was able to do at work in a chair. We waited a full three months before graduating to Core Routine I (page 62), which Chuck then practiced at least twice a week.

After three months, Chuck had noticed a significant difference in how he felt. His energy was returning, and his exercise tolerance was steadily increasing. At six months he reported that his stress level had dropped remarkably. His cholesterol level also decreased so much that his doctor lowered the dosage of his medication. After a year, Chuck was thrilled to be able to resume snow skiing with his family, and he has avoided any further heart attacks. After five years, Chuck is still practicing Yoga, and recently his cardiologist gave him his best report ever on a heart exam.

When it comes to cardiovascular disorders, Yoga is no longer considered an "alternative" treatment. Doctors now routinely recommend it to heart patients, along with other gentle mind–body practices such as Tai Chi and biofeedback. The physical practice of Yoga and the lifestyle changes inherent in the Yoga philosophy work together to calm your heart and mind, bring your circulatory system back into balance, and help you avoid the number-one killer of Americans today: heart disease.

ANATOMY 101

The Circulatory System

The circulatory system consists of the heart and the blood vessels. The heart pumps blood into the arteries, which supply the body with oxygenated blood and nutrients. The blood returns from the organs back to the heart through the veins.

The circulatory system has many purposes including the following:

- Capturing oxygen from the lungs and delivering it to the whole body.
- Getting food nutrients from the gastrointestinal system (stomach and intestines) and delivering them throughout the body.
- Circulating hormones around the body.
- Removing carbon dioxide, which is a waste product, and taking it to the lungs where it can be released through exhalation.
- Getting rid of other waste products by running the blood through the kidneys and liver.

The circulatory system works well when the heart pumps efficiently, not too hard or soft, not too fast or slow, allowing the blood vessels to deliver blood to where it needs to go and to return it back to the heart. Heart failure occurs when, for a variety of reasons, the heart cannot effectively pump blood.

CIRCULATORY AILMENTS

Hypertension

Hypertension, also known as high blood pressure, affects a quarter of all American adults and fully half of those over the age of sixty. Health-care professionals attribute the pervasiveness of this disease to the U.S. lifestyle of excess: smoking, too much alcohol, too much cholesterol and fat, too much salt, too much stress, and too much body weight. Add to this the consequences of not enough exercise, and you can see why many of us are living our lives on the edge.

Blood pressure refers to the amount of pressure in your arteries, which changes with each pump of your heart. Hypertension occurs when the pressure in the system gets high enough to start causing problems in your body. Conditions that cause the blood pressure to rise are usually related to the blood vessels being either constricted or overfilled; in both cases, it takes more force to pump the blood through them.

When blood pressure rises above normal, the blood's normal pulsating is replaced by a pounding. Even a very slight rise in blood pressure is significant, when you consider that the heart beats over one hundred thousand times per day. This relentless battering is very hard on the walls of the blood vessels and weakens them. The high pressure can also cause damage to various organs: In the kidneys the excess pressure can damage the vessels that filter waste products from the blood, making the kidneys ineffective and leading to kidney failure.[1] In the brain, a type of stroke can result when the damaged vessels rupture. Stroke is the third leading cause of death in the United States (after heart disease and cancer), and high blood pressure is the main risk factor.[2] In the heart, the hammering damages the arterial linings, hastening cholesterol buildup that can lead to heart attack. Uncontrolled hypertension also causes the heart muscle itself to work harder and eventually lose its ability to pump effectively, a condition that can lead to congestive heart failure.

In the last few decades of the twentieth century, very effective medications were developed to control blood pressure, and they've greatly reduced the number of deaths directly attributed to hypertension. But since taking medication does not address the root causes of high blood pressure, cardiovascular specialists and primary-care physicians usually prescribe lifestyle changes first, especially for people whose blood pressure is only slightly elevated. Behavioral adjustments are recommended even for those taking hypertension drugs, because if carried out, modifications in diet and exercise levels can reduce or eliminate the need for medication.[3] If you have been diagnosed with hypertension, be sure to read The Yoga Prescription for Circulatory Ailments on page 179 and Yoga for Hypertension on page 182.

Coronary Artery Disease

Coronary artery disease (CAD) is the most common form of heart disease. Sometimes called ischemic heart disease, it results when the coronary arteries—the fuel lines leading into and out of the heart—are clogged with plaque. The plaque is made of cholesterol, fat, calcium, blood clots, and other debris.[4] This leads to a number of problems:

- Angina (pain, pressure, or burning in the chest, neck, or arm)
- Irregular heart rhythms (mild to life threatening)
- Breathlessness, fatigue, and loss of tolerance for exertion
- Congestive heart failure
- Heart attack
- Death

The clogging of the arteries begins when the arterial walls are damaged, by the battering force of high blood pressure, by toxic substances entering the body through cigarettes and fatty foods, or by excess adrenaline flowing through the bloodstream because of stress.

Once the arterial wall is damaged, the buildup starts. This is a long, slow process called atherosclerosis that can begin in youth and continue for decades. The plaque is deposited, layer upon layer, making the interior of the arteries smaller and smaller. The crisis occurs when something, usually a blood clot or a piece of the unstable plaque, completely blocks the flow of blood. If this causes a portion of the heart muscle to die, it is called a myocardial infarction, or a heart attack.

The progression of CAD can be so gradual and the symptoms so variable that in half of all people with CAD, the very first symptom is death.[5] According to recent polls, most women believe that they are most likely to die of breast cancer, but heart disease claims six times as many women.[6] If you have been diagnosed with heart disease or CAD, be sure to read The Yoga Prescription for Circulatory Ailments on page 179 and Yoga for Heart Disease and Coronary Artery Disease on page 188.

The Yoga Advantage for Circulatory Ailments

Doreen is a forty-seven-year-old school teacher in Los Angeles. After seventeen years at the grammar-school level, she accepted a higher-paying position in an inner-city high school. A year later she discovered she had high blood pressure, and for the next five years was on daily hypertension medication. She had side effects from the medicine, but each time she stopped taking it, her blood pressure would spike back up again. Doreen was depressed about her situation and began consultation with a psychologist, who referred her to me.

On our first visit I learned that Doreen was about twenty pounds overweight and was having frequent nightmares. She ate a lot of salty foods and often watched the local news just before bed. I recommended a low-salt, low-fat, vegetarian diet and referred her to Dr. Dean Ornish's book *Eat More, Weigh Less*. She began daily practice of a Yoga routine designed for people with hypertension, and a separate Yoga breathing practice for her afternoon break, right after the end of the school day. She incorporated a simple walking program three to five days a week, beginning with ten minutes and gradually increasing to thirty, and replaced the evening news with a relaxation technique or a few pages from a good book.

After two months of her new way of life, Doreen's physician reduced her blood pressure medicine by half. By the end of the third month she had lost fifteen pounds and was able to discontinue her medication completely. Doreen truly feels like a new person. Her depression has lifted, she maintains a normal weight, and her blood pressure has been normal for more than a year without any medication.

There are a few risk factors for circulatory ailments that we have no control over, such as our family history and our age. However, most of the conditions leading to hypertension and heart disease are within our power to regulate: smoking, the amount of fat and salt in our diet, our weight, how much we exercise, and how much stress we deal with in our lives. Each of these factors affects the state of our blood vessels, determining the health of our organs and our risk of cardiovascular problems. Following the Yoga lifestyle for wellness described in Chapter 1 can help us to overcome many harmful practices. Research has shown that circulatory problems respond well to various Yoga regimens, from a few simple postures performed twice a week to a complete overhaul of lifestyle practices.

A number of reputable studies have established the benefit of using Yoga to treat high blood pressure. A classic study done in 1969 showed that the daily use of just one posture, the Corpse (described later in this chapter), significantly reduced blood pressure after only three weeks.[7] In another study, twenty-five hypertension patients were given Yoga therapy, and after six months all showed a significant decrease in blood pressure. Five of the patients had been taking hypertension medicine, and all were able to decrease their dosage.[8] In a study published in 2000, half of the participants practiced an hour of Yoga twice daily, and the other half received drug treatment. After eleven weeks, the researchers noted that Yoga was as effective as the medication in controlling hypertension.[9] Several studies have shown that stress reduction through various behavioral procedures such as Yoga, biofeedback, meditation, and psychotherapy benefit hypertension patients by lowering their blood pressure.[10]

In 1990, the International Association of Yoga Therapists (IAYT) conducted a three-month study on Yoga and hypertension. The postures used in this pilot study were similar to those I used for my client Doreen (see Yoga for Hypertension on page 182). The subjects in the study changed nothing in their lifestyle except for adding the Yoga routine, yet their blood pressure decreased a statistically significant 6.5 percent.[11]

Dr. Ornish is well known for his pioneering work in the reversal of heart disease. One of his most famous studies, published in 1998, showed that lifestyle changes can be even more effective than medication for treating coronary artery disease.[12] Additional studies have verified the benefits of a healthy lifestyle for heart patients, and researchers have gone even further to show that adding Yoga can have a profound impact. One study involved two groups of men with CAD. One group was put on a program of diet and risk-factor control. The other group was given the same diet and risk-factor control program but was also prescribed daily Yoga practice and moderate aerobic exercise. After a year, the Yoga group had better exercise capacity, lower body weight, and significantly fewer bypass surgeries and other medical interventions than the other group.[13] The researchers attributed the improvement to the combined effects of Yoga, exercise, and diet. Another study conducted in India examined two groups of heart patients. One group was taught Yoga four days a week and was encouraged to practice at home in between classes. After only fourteen weeks, the Yoga practitioners showed markedly greater improvement in measures of heart disease.[14]

Adding a Yoga routine to your schedule can have tremendous benefits for your cardiovascular health. But why is this true? One of the main reasons is that the stress you allow into your mind is a key player in hypertension. The calming nature of Yoga, particularly breathing exercises, relaxation techniques, and meditation, can transform your experience of the pressures of everyday living. Many type-A personalities find particular refuge in Yoga relaxation techniques.

Yoga's effect on our circulatory health has been explained by the work of Herbert Benson, the Harvard physician we discussed earlier in the book. His research focused on the physiology of our relaxation response. He found that the relaxation breathing we practice in Yoga stimulates the parasympathetic nervous system, which is responsible for telling our bodies to relax. This in turn reduces the heart rate and the intensity of the heart pump, thereby lowering blood pressure.

Light to moderate aerobic exercise is usually recommended as part of a heart-healthy routine, even for those with circulatory ailments, and our overall Yoga prescription for cardiovascular health includes that advice. Yet it is important to note the differences in how Yoga and aerobic exercise affect your heart. Workouts consisting of jogging, running, and other fast-paced aerobics bring more blood flow to the heart while raising your heart rate, pulse, blood pressure, and oxygen consumption. These exercises can be very good for the heart, lungs, muscles, and blood vessels. If you exercise too intensely, and the oxygen demand is greater than your body's ability to supply the oxygen to your muscles, then waste products such as lactic acid begin to build up in your muscles. In contrast, Yoga postures and breathing exercises are gentle aerobic exercises that do not outpace your body's ability to supply oxygen to the heart and other muscles. At the end of a Yoga session, you feel refreshed. In addition, your mind is quiet and calm, which is not usually the case after an hour of working out to loud music in an aerobics or spinning class. We recommend that you work with your doctor to establish an exercise plan that combines an aerobic activity such as walking, swimming, or cycling with a daily Yoga routine.

Practicing Yoga can also help you control other risk factors for heart problems. For example, many people mistakenly believe that smoking or overeating helps them relax or deal with stress. As Dr. Benson demonstrated, the relaxation response that results from Yoga breathing can calm your nervous system, decreasing your cravings, and giving you a greater sense of control over what you put in your body. Richard Usatine and other physicians routinely use Yoga breathing to help patients quit smoking. Dr. Usatine recommends that while you are in the process of quitting smoking, you should take a Yoga Breathing Break whenever you are feeling stress, anxiety, or craving for a cigarette. After a short period of Yoga breathing, you should be able to go on without reaching for a deadly cigarette.

Medications used to treat heart disease and hypertension sometimes have unpleasant side effects. One of the greatest advantages of Yoga is that it can treat circulatory problems without side effects, and it can decrease or eliminate the need for medication. For the millions in the United States who are taking daily medicine for heart problems, this is good news.

The Yoga Prescription for Circulatory Ailments

- Add physical activity to your daily life, particularly light to moderate aerobic exercise such as walking.
- If you are overweight, losing just ten pounds can lower your blood pressure up to 30 percent.

- Decrease the salt in your diet as much as possible. Read food labels to detect such ingredients as salt, soda, or sodium. While not all hypertension will decrease with a low-salt diet, if it seems to improve your blood pressure readings, then it is important you continue limiting your sodium. A home blood pressure monitor may help you determine how your blood pressure responds to a lower salt intake and other lifestyle changes.

- Eat a high-fiber diet, which helps reduce cholesterol levels. Include oat bran and whole grains such as brown rice, buckwheat, millet, and oats.

- Eat plenty of fresh fruits and vegetables. The American Dietetic Association recommends at least five servings per day.

- Keep your fat intake under control if you have high cholesterol. Fish and poultry are acceptable in moderation, but avoid fatty red meat. The best way to minimize fat intake from fish, poultry, and meat is to trim away the skin and visible pieces of fat. Using fat-free dairy products and eating smaller food portions overall can help keep your fat intake under control.

- Alcohol and caffeine should be used in moderation. While small amounts of caffeine or alcohol (such as one cup or glass per day) may be safe, too much can raise your blood pressure.

- Do not use any tobacco products (cigarettes, cigars, chewing tobacco). There is no safe level of use for any of these. Even secondhand smoke can be dangerous to your heart, lungs, and blood vessels.

- Get plenty of sleep. If you wake up groggy in the morning or need large doses of caffeine to get you through the day, you're not getting enough rest.

- Take steps to manage your stress. Learn Yoga breathing techniques (see Chapter 4) so that they are at your disposal whenever you need them. Incorporate a Yoga Breathing Break into your regular schedule, at the time of day when you are usually most stressed.

- If you're taking hypertension medication, discuss your new Yoga program with your doctor. Measure your own blood pressure or get regular checkups to determine if your dosage can be reduced or the medication eliminated.

- Stay involved with other people. Consider clubs, exercise classes, or activities with organizations that represent your faith. Volunteering to work with a charitable association is a great way to be involved with other people and to contribute to your community. Numerous studies show that lonely, depressed, or isolated people are much more likely to die prematurely.

❋ Practice the appropriate Yoga routine from this chapter. Start with two or three days a week, working toward five to six days a week.

YOGA FOR CIRCULATORY AILMENTS

Yoga for Hypertension

This program is the one I created for my client Doreen (page 176) for her hypertension. If your blood pressure is not controlled (higher than 140/90 mm Hg with or without medication) or if you have any uncontrolled heart disease, be sure to talk with your physician before starting. This routine takes approximately fifteen minutes, and should be practiced using Focused Breathing (page 39). Ideally, practice the routine twice a day until your condition improves, then practice it once a day. When you feel your condition has subsided, you may cut down to three times a week.

Seated Posture

This simple relaxing posture supports and stabilizes the spine, facilitating good sitting posture.

1. Sit comfortably in an armless chair, bringing your body slightly away from the back rest.
2. Let your arms hang down by your sides. Place your feet evenly on the floor at hip width. If your feet do not touch the floor, place a folded blanket or a phone book under them. Your thighs should be parallel to the floor, with your knees and hips bent at approximately a 90 degree angle.
3. Place your hands on your thighs with your fingers toward your knees. Bring your back up nice and tall, and gently pull your head back until your ears, shoulders, and hip sockets are in alignment. Do not force anything beyond your comfort level.
4. Use Focused Breathing (page 39) for 8 to 10 breaths. Gently draw the belly in on the exhale.

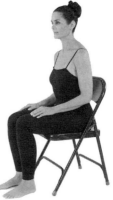

Seated Arm Raise

This movement improves the range of motion of and increases blood flow to the upper back and shoulders.

1. Start in the Seated Posture.
2. Let your arms hang at your sides, palms turned back. Look straight ahead.
3. As you inhale, raise your arms forward and up overhead.
4. As you exhale, bring your arms back down as in Step 2.
5. Repeat slowly, 4 to 6 times.

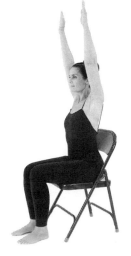

Standing Forward Bend with Chair

This gentle stretch promotes circulation in the upper torso and head. It stretches the entire back of the body, including the neck, shoulders, hamstrings, and back.

Caution: If you have been diagnosed with an intervertebral disk problem, be careful of all forward bends. Avoid this posture if it causes back pain. Check with your physician or other health-care professional if you are uncertain.

1. Stand with your feet hip-width apart, arm's distance from the seat of a chair. Keep the spine tall but relaxed. Let your arms hang at your sides, palms turned inward toward your legs. Look straight ahead.
2. As you inhale, raise your arms to the front, up and overhead.
3. As you exhale, slowly bend forward from the hips, bringing your arms, hands, torso, and head forward and down until your palms touch the front edge of the chair. Slightly bend your knees.
4. As you inhale, return to the upright position, keeping your arms raised.
5. Repeat 3 times. Then stay in the forward bend position for 6 to 8 breaths. Slowly return to an upright position.

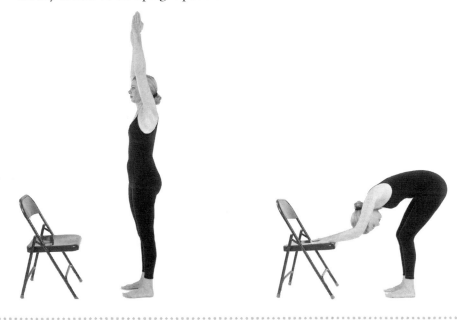

Sitting Cat

This posture relaxes and gently stretches the lower and upper back. (If you have knee or hip problems, replace Sitting Cat with Knees to Chest, described on page 186. Thus you will be doing Knees to Chest twice in this routine.)

1. Start on your hands and knees, looking slightly down, with the heels of your hands directly below your shoulders and the knees at hip width.
2. As you exhale, sit back on your heels and bring your head toward the floor. Work toward resting your torso on your thighs with your forehead on the floor, but do not force it. Sit back only as far as comfortable.
3. Repeat 3 times, and then relax with your head down and your arms in front (as in Step 2), for 6 to 8 breaths.

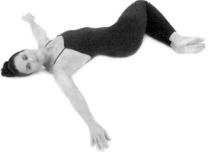

Lying Bent-Legs Twist

This gentle twisting motion tones the abdomen, exercises the spine, and has a calming effect on the nervous system.

1. Lie flat on your back with your knees bent and feet on the floor at hip width. Move your arms out from your sides in a T, aligned with the tops of your shoulders, palms down.
2. As you exhale, slowly lower your bent legs to the right side; then turn your head to the left. It is important to keep your head on the floor.
3. As you inhale, bring your bent legs back to the middle. Exhale, while slowly lowering your bent legs to the left side. Turn your head to the right.
4. Alternating sides, repeat slowly 3 times to each side. Hold the last twist to each side for 6 to 8 breaths.

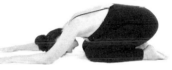

Knees to Chest

This slow stretching motion relieves stiffness and discomfort in the lower back. We also use it for balance after a twist. (Note that Knees to Chest is different from Knee to Chest, which appears elsewhere in the book.)

1. Lie on your back with your knees bent, feet on the floor at hip width. Bring your bent knees toward your chest and hold on to the top of your shins, just below your knees, one hand on each knee. If you are having knee problems, hold the backs of your thighs, under your knees.
2. As you exhale, draw your knees toward your chest. As you inhale, move the knees a few inches away from your chest, rolling your hips to the floor.
3. Repeat 3 times, and then stay in the most folded position for 6 to 8 breaths. Slowly return your feet to the floor in the bent-knee position.

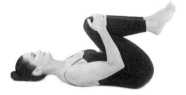

Legs on a Chair with Eyes Covered

This relaxation technique uses a chair to improve circulation to your legs, hips, and lower back. It has a calming effect on your nervous system.

1. Place a chair in an area where you have room to lie down in front of it.
2. Lie on your back with knees bent, feet on the floor. The front edge of the chair's seat should be turned toward you, just in front of your feet.
3. Lift your feet off the floor and lay your calves on the chair seat, with the front edge of the seat tucked into the backs of your knees. Cover your eyes with an eye bag or small folded towel. If your head tilts back, place a blanket under it.
4. Inhale freely, then gradually increase the length of your exhalation over several breaths until you reach your comfortable maximum. Continue with the long exhalation for 3 to 5 minutes. When finished, gradually bring the breath back to normal and sit for 2 or 3 minutes before standing.

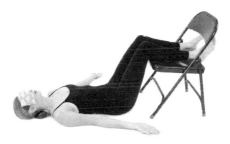

Breathing Break

Use Alternate Nostril Breathing (page 45) for 3 to 5 minutes.

Yoga for Heart Disease
and Coronary Artery Disease

If you've been diagnosed with heart disease or CAD, you can immediately benefit from practicing this single Yoga posture, two or three times a day. You may eventually be able to graduate to a full Yoga routine.

....

Corpse (Supported) with Eyes Covered

This is the safest and most popular Yoga posture, a classic for relaxation of the body and mind. It soothes the nervous system and facilitates deep rest.

1. Lie on your back. Place a bolster, pillows, or folded blankets under your upper back for support. Your arms should be relaxed near your sides, palms turned up. Cover your eyes with an eye bag or folded towel. If your head tilts back or your neck is uncomfortable, place a small pillow or blanket under your head and neck. If your lower back is uncomfortable, place a pillow or rolled blanket under your knees. You may also do the Corpse without supports.
2. Relax for 5 to 15 minutes, using Belly Breathing with Long Exhalation (page 136).

It's important that you work closely with your physician to determine when you're ready to move beyond the Corpse to begin practicing a complete Yoga routine. Here's what to do when you are ready:

* Begin with the Lower Back Routine (page 114).
* Add the Neck and Upper Back Routine (page 129) when you feel comfortable.
* Graduate to Core Routine I (page 62).

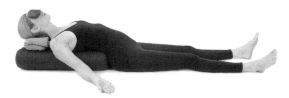

....

10

The Digestive System: Irritable Bowel

Syndrome, Heartburn

In Chapter 8 we discussed the ancient Yoga philosophy that breath equals life. Here in the West, many of us would be more likely to say that *food* equals life. In our culture, the enjoyment of food is a top priority, far more important than its nutritional value. Major celebrations are centered around eating. Fast-food joints and swanky restaurants are everywhere. Our pantries and freezers are stocked to the brim, and still we want our pizza delivered in half an hour or less. So when something goes wrong with our body's ability to efficiently process the food we eat, it can be enormously distressing.

I met Alicia, a thirty-eight-year-old artist and mother, at the Esalen Institute in Big Sur, California, while I was teaching a weekend Yoga seminar. Fifteen minutes before our class began, she was already in the room pacing the floor and expressing numerous worries about the difficulty of the class. I invited her to sit for a few minutes and get acquainted.

She explained that she had suffered from numerous digestive problems since becoming a mother seven years earlier. She had been hospitalized several times with irritable bowel syndrome (IBS) and frequently experienced acid reflux. Much to her disappointment, I recommended against the group class until I could spend some time with her, since several Yoga postures are problematic for IBS and acid reflux. We met twice more that weekend and I learned that Alicia had used a great deal of medication to treat her symptoms but had never considered trying to get to the cause of her ailments. I arranged some counseling referrals near her home and created a conservative Yoga program for her to practice on her own, similar to the one in this chapter for IBS and acid reflux. The program emphasizes calming the nervous system, gently massaging the intestines and stomach, and increasing circulation to the area. We avoided any inverted postures, prone postures (lying on the belly), or postures that put pressure on the abdominal area. When she returned home, Alicia started psychotherapy and nutritional counseling, and began practicing her Yoga routine regularly. I taught her what to avoid in a group class and how to substitute postures she could do for ones that were inappropriate for her conditions. After three months, Alicia told me that the combination of Yoga, diet, and counseling have reduced her suffering dramatically. She is elated that her IBS and acid reflux have calmed down, saying, "I'm much less anxious on a daily basis, and even my friends have noticed a difference in my moods and temperament."

Digestive ailments such as Alicia's can be awful to deal with and difficult to talk about. Sometimes it seems easier to take a bunch of medicine and hope for the best, rather than find a way to really solve the problem. But Yoga has a long tradition of healing these disorders. In fact, Yoga philosophy contends that the abdomen is the seat of sickness and wellness; therefore many of the postures of Yoga were designed specifically to enhance abdominal health.

The Yogis' view of the significance of the digestive system is also reflected in the ancient Sanskrit word for food, *anna,* which has two seemingly opposite meanings: "that which nourishes you" or "that which lives on you, or kills you."[1] If you suffer from digestive ailments, you know exactly how both meanings can be true. While these disorders are not necessarily *caused* by food, they can change your experience of eating from gratifying to unpleasant or even downright dangerous.

ANATOMY 101

The Digestive System

The digestive system consists of approximately thirty-three feet of plumbing that begins at your mouth and ends at your rectum. The best way to understand it is to take a journey through it from the point of view of a piece of food. The food enters your mouth, where digestive juices from saliva begin to break it down into more usable molecules to provide nutrients to your organs and cells. Your teeth mash up the food to make it easier to swallow and more readily available to the salivary enzymes. You then swallow the food, and it travels down the esophagus with the help of gravity and peristalsis. (Peristalsis is a contracting motion that occurs all along the digestive tract to help move food along.) The food lands in your stomach where various digestive juices break it down further. The stomach pushes the food into the duodenum, which is the beginning of the small intestine. In the stomach and duodenum, the acid is highly concentrated. Therefore these regions are the most common areas for ulcers and acid-related problems. As the food passes through the duodenum, your pancreas delivers its special digestive enzymes which help process sugars. Your liver also sends a unique chemical called bile, which is used for fat digestion. (The gallbladder stores the bile and can deliver it into the small intestine, but since your liver can do this without the gallbladder, the gallbladder is not an essential organ.)

The food continues to move along the long narrow tube that we call the small intestine. While there, the essential nutrients of the food get absorbed into the bloodstream and pass through the liver for detoxification. The sugars, carbohydrates, proteins, and fats are absorbed into the bloodstream through the small intestine, to be transferred throughout the body via the circulatory system. Whatever food does not get absorbed into the bloodstream will pass into the large intestine, which has a larger diameter than the small intestine but is significantly shorter. The job of the large intestine, also called the colon or the bowels, is to remove the extra water out of the remaining waste products so that your bowel movements will not be excessively watery. This helps your body conserve water and produce a formed stool. Both within the medical community and without, you often see the terms digestive system, intestines, and bowels used synonymously.

DIGESTIVE AILMENTS

Irritable Bowel Syndrome

The most common gastrointestinal disorder is IBS. Approximately one out of six Americans experience it, and a quarter of them see a physician because of their symptoms. Though it can affect just about anybody, the most common sufferers are between the ages of fifteen and forty-five, with females being affected more than males.[2]

IBS is a disorder of the intestines that leads to crampy pain, gassiness, bloating, and changes in bowel habits. IBS can cause you to have constipation, diarrhea, or alternate between the two. Through the years, this disorder has been called by many names, such as colitis, mucous colitis, spastic colon, and spastic bowel. These are all laypeople's terms for IBS, but none of them is really accurate. IBS can cause a great deal of suffering and anxiety, but it does *not* cause permanent harm to the intestines and does not lead to any serious illness. Doctors call it a functional disorder because there is no inflammation or sign of disease when the intestines are examined. It is not to be confused with ulcerative colitis, however, which is a different disorder that is more severe and involves inflammation in the colon.[3]

In healthy people, eating causes contractions of the colon, which may cause an urge to have a bowel movement within an hour after a meal. (This is called the gastrocolic reflex.) In people with IBS, the urge often comes sooner and with a vengeance—accompanied by cramps and diarrhea.

Certain medicines and foods may trigger intestinal spasms in some sufferers of IBS. Sometimes the spasm leads to constipation. Chocolate, milk products, and large amounts of alcohol are frequent offenders. Caffeine may cause loose stools in healthy people, but it is more likely to affect those with IBS.

Before changing your diet, it is a good idea to keep a journal, noting which foods or patterns of eating seem to cause distress. You may want to consult a registered dietitian, who can help you make changes in your diet. And be sure to discuss your findings with your doctor.

Researchers have found that women with IBS may have more symptoms during their menstrual periods, suggesting that reproductive hormones can increase IBS symptoms. Other contributing factors may include inadequate time on the toilet to relax the bowels and lack of exercise.[4] Most people with IBS are able to control their symptoms through diet, exercise, stress management, and medication prescribed by their physician.

Heartburn

Gastroesophageal reflux disease (GERD) is the medical term for what we commonly call heartburn or acid indigestion. More than sixty million American adults experience heartburn at least once a month, and about twenty-five million adults suffer from it daily. Although GERD can be uncomfortable to the point of limiting daily activities and productivity, it is rarely life threatening.[5]

Gastroesophageal reflux literally means "the return of the stomach's contents back up into the esophagus." The disorder affects the lower esophageal sphincter (LES)—the muscle connecting the esophagus with the stomach. In normal digestion, the LES opens to allow food to pass into the stomach, and closes to prevent food and acidic stomach juices from flowing back into the esophagus. Reflux occurs when the LES is weak or relaxes inappropriately, allowing the stomach's contents to flow back up.

Sri Mishra, M.D., associate professor of neurology at the University of Southern California School of Medicine and a Yoga expert, says he attributes digestive problems such as GERD to the "hurry, worry, and curry" syndrome. In other words: stress, anxiety, and the wrong foods. Doctors recommend lifestyle and dietary changes for most people with GERD. Certain foods and beverages, including chocolate, fried or fatty foods, coffee, and alcoholic beverages may open the LES, causing reflux and heartburn. In addition, some foods can irritate a damaged esophageal lining, such as citrus fruits and juices, tomato products, and pepper. All of these problem foods should be avoided. Decreasing the size of portions at mealtime may also help control symptoms. Always avoid lying down immediately after eating any meal or snack. Eating meals at least two to three hours before bedtime may lessen reflux by allowing the acid in the stomach to decrease and the stomach to empty before going to bed.

Studies show that cigarette smoking weakens the LES. Therefore, stopping smoking is an important way to reduce GERD symptoms. In addition, being overweight often worsens symptoms, and many overweight people find relief when they lose weight.

Stress is a major contributor to heartburn. People usually find that when they reduce their stress through Yoga postures and relaxation techniques, their heartburn decreases. The right Yoga postures can also soothe the abdominal area and help prevent GERD.

The Yoga Advantage for Digestive Ailments

According to the Bihar School of Yoga, the solution to digestive problems lies in elevating the eating process from a mechanical habit to a conscious and pleasurable act, in which moderate quantities of simple pure food are eaten with full awareness. This is an ideal unlikely to be met at all times, especially in our fast-paced, eat-on-the-run society. Fortunately, even a small improvement in your diet, combined with a Yoga practice and some stress relief, will likely improve your digestive problems.

Roger was a 42-year-old money manager with a high-profile, high-maintenance client base—and a high-stress, fast-track lifestyle to go with it. He burned the candle at both ends, and ate indiscriminately. He dealt with his chronic symptoms of heartburn by consuming massive amounts of over-the-counter antacids. Because he remained slender regardless of his diet, he rationalized that he did not need to exercise and bragged that he never saw a doctor. His wife asked him to try Yoga but he was too busy and was sure he didn't need it.

One afternoon, after a weekend of little sleep, a lot of spicy food, and the loss of one of his major clients, his heartburn got so bad that his medications did not help and he feared he was having a heart attack. He described the pain as though "someone was shoving the heel of their foot into his heart." Because he had no doctor to call, his wife took him to a crowded emergency room where he truly thought he was going to die. After being treated with stronger medications and subjected to numerous tests, he was assured that he was not having a heart attack. The treating doctor cautioned Roger, however, that unless he wanted to repeat this ordeal, he had to change his diet and lifestyle, and recommended Yoga. This time he listened. Referred by his wife and one of his clients, he came to me for Yoga therapy. He felt tremendous improvement after only one session in which he learned a routine similar to the one in this chapter. He went home with it on audiotape and the suggestions that he avoid spicy foods and stop eating at least three hours before sleeping. Happily, Roger made a quick turn-around. After three months he was off of his medicines completely and much calmer in his work and home life.

The ancient Yogis use the image of *agni*—Sanskrit for "fire"—to understand the power of digestion. In this theory, digestive disorders reflect some imbalance in the internal fire. With GERD and IBS, the digestive fire is too strong, and these are called hyperagni conditions.[6]

When using Yoga to treat hyperagni conditions, such as heartburn and irritable bowel syndrome, we need to soothe the digestive system, not strain it. Dr. Mishra encourages gentle folding and twisting postures for heartburn and IBS. He also recommends relaxation and meditation for these ailments, since stress is such a large factor.

The Yoga Prescription for Digestive Ailments

❋ If you take a group Yoga class, be sure you are with a qualified instructor. Talk with the instructor before the class, to learn which postures you may need to avoid.

❋ Try to establish the habit of early morning evacuation of the bowels. It is best to wait until after breakfast, when the gastrocolic reflex should aid the process of evacuation.

❋ Improve your diet, making sure to include plenty of fiber and fluids and staying away from foods that seem to aggravate your condition.

❋ Do regular cardiovascular exercise such as brisk walking, swimming, or cycling, but not right after eating. Your circulation is needed to digest your food, and should not be competing with the muscles during exercise.

❋ Try to develop self-awareness while eating, a fundamental Yoga practice. Be regular with meal times and eat slowly. Try to extract maximum pleasure from each morsel rather than unconsciously stuffing yourself. Don't eat when you are anxious or tense.

❋ Practice the Yoga therapy routine from this chapter. Start with two or three days a week, working toward five or six days a week.

Tips for Heartburn

✳ Avoid foods and beverages that affect the LES or irritate the esophagus lining, including fried and fatty foods, chocolate, alcohol, coffee, citrus fruits and juices, and tomato products. (Some people with heartburn can tolerate these foods. Use your own judgment and pass up the ones that activate your symptoms.)

✳ Lose a few pounds if you are overweight.

✳ Don't smoke.

✳ Avoid lying down for two to three hours after eating.

YOGA FOR DIGESTIVE AILMENTS

Yoga for Irritable Bowel Syndrome and Heartburn

This program is similar to the one I gave to Alicia (page 189) for her IBS and heartburn. It takes approximately fifteen minutes and should be practiced using Focused Breathing (page 39). Try to inhale and exhale through your nose, pausing briefly after the inhalation and the exhalation. Ideally, practice the routine twice a day until your condition improves, then practice it once a day. When you feel your condition has subsided, you may cut down to three times a week.

Supported Easy Posture

This opening posture increases the flexibility of your hips and spine, and prepares you for more advanced sitting postures. A blanket adds comfort and supports the natural curves of your spine.

1   Sit on the floor with a folded blanket under your hips for comfort. Cross your legs at your ankles, left leg on top, right leg on the bottom. (Alternate from day to day.)

2. Press your palms down on the floor while you move each foot toward the opposite knee as far as possible. Ideally, your right foot will be underneath your left knee, and your left foot underneath your right knee, but don't force it.

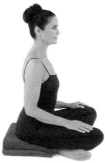

3. Bring your head and spine up nice and tall with a slight lift in your chest until your ear, shoulder, and hip are in vertical alignment. Place your hands comfortably on your knees with your elbows bent. Stay in this posture for 8 to 10 breaths.

Flowing Cat and Dog Sequence

This exercise gently compresses and stretches your abdomen. The use of the soft sounds *ah* and *ma* soothe your belly. The sequence also relaxes and gently stretches your lower and upper back, neck, and shoulders.

1. Kneel upright with your knees at hip width and your arms at your sides.
2. As you inhale, raise your arms from the front up and overhead until your arms and ears are in alignment and your palms are facing in.
3. Exhale, using the sound *ah* as you bend forward, moving your hips back toward your heels and placing your head, arms, and palms on the floor. Sit back only as far as comfortable.
4. As you inhale, move your chest and head forward, gently arching your back, and raise your head slightly.
5. As you exhale, use the sound *ma* and sit back again as in Step 3.
6. As you inhale, raise up to the upright kneeling position with your arms overhead as in Step 1. Repeat Steps 1 to 5 in a continuous flow 4 to 6 times. Be sure to use the sounds *ah* and *ma* on the exhale.

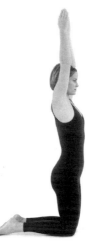

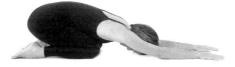

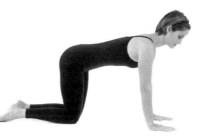

Seated Chair Twist

This posture gently compresses and twists your stomach and intestines, promoting better circulation.

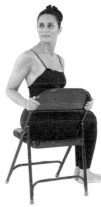

1. Sit sideways on a chair with the chair back to your right, feet flat on the floor, and heels directly below the knees.
2. Exhale, turn to the right, and grasp the sides of the chair back with your hands. If your feet are not comfortably on the floor, place a folded blanket or a phone book under them.
3. As you inhale, bring your back up tall, as if you were trying to touch the ceiling with the top of your spine.
4. As you exhale, twist your torso and head farther to the right.
5. Return to the starting position. Repeat the twist, gradually twisting farther with each exhalation for 3 breaths, but do not go beyond your comfort zone. On the last repetition, hold the twist for 4 to 6 breaths.
6. Repeat the same sequence on the opposite side.

Sitting Fold

This posture gently compresses and stretches your abdominal area. It also gives a nice stretch to your hips and lower back.

1. Sit sideways on a chair with the chair back to your left, feet flat on the floor. Place your heels directly below your knees. Put your hands on your thighs with your fingers facing forward, near your knees.
2. As you exhale, bend forward from your hips and slide your hands forward and down your legs. Hang your head and arms down and relax briefly in the folded position.
3. As you inhale, roll your torso, head, and arms back up to the initial seated position.
4. Repeat slowly 4 to 6 times.

Lying Bent-Legs Twist

This twist gently compresses and twists your stomach and your intestines, promoting better circulation.

1. Lie flat on your back with your knees bent and feet on the floor at hip width. Move your arms out from your sides in a T, aligned with the tops of your shoulders, palms down.
2. As you exhale, slowly lower your bent legs to the right side; then turn your head to the left. It is important to keep your head on the floor.
3. As you inhale, bring your bent legs back to the middle. Exhale, while slowly lowering your bent legs to the left side. Turn your head to the right.

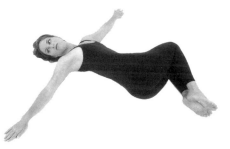

4. Alternating sides, repeat slowly 3 times to each side. Hold the last twist to each side for 6 to 8 breaths. Return your feet to the floor in the bent knee position.

Knees to Chest

This gentle stretch compresses your stomach and your intestines and relieves abdominal gas. It also compensates your lower back after a twisting posture.

1. Lie on your back with your knees bent, feet on the floor at hip width. Bring your bent knees toward your chest and hold on to the top of your shins, just below your knees, one hand on each knee. If you are having knee problems, hold the backs of your thighs, under your knees.
2. As you exhale, draw your knees toward your chest. As you inhale, move your knees a few inches away from your chest, rolling your hips to the floor.
3. Repeat 3 times, and then stay in the most folded position for 6 to 8 breaths.

Corpse (Supported) with Belly Breathing

This is the classic posture for relaxation of the body and mind. It gives a gentle opening to your chest and brings circulation to the gastric area and reduces acidity.

1. Lie flat on your back with your arms at your sides, palms up. Place blankets under your upper back to gently open your chest. Place blankets or pillows under your head and neck for support. Cover your eyes if you like. If the supported position doesn't feel right to you, lie flat on your back in the classic Corpse.
2. Practice Belly Breathing (page 41), gradually increasing the length of your exhalation until you reach your comfortable maximum. Repeat for 8 to 10 breaths.

Relaxation or Meditation

1. Stay in the Corpse (Supported) position.
2. Practice Yoga Nidra (page 53) or Focused Meditation (page 57) for at least five minutes.

Breathing Break

Once per day, use Victorious Breath (page 44) or Belly Breathing (page 41) with long exhalation for three to five minutes.

11

The Nervous System:

Tension Headaches, Migraines

Sometimes it seems our modern society has perfected the art of stress-filled living, but we certainly didn't invent the headache. People have been suffering them throughout recorded history, and ancient Yoga literature is filled with mentions of headaches and Yoga strategies for handling them.

Headache is one of the most universal human ailments. Most everybody gets one now and then, and there are millions who suffer from chronic, even daily headaches. It is estimated that twenty-six million people in this country are afflicted with migraines.[1] While many systems of the body can be involved in headaches, it is the nervous system that is primarily responsible for the pain.

NEUROSCIENCE 101

The Nervous System

Your nervous system includes the brain, the spinal cord, and the nerves that radiate into all parts of your body. This system commands and coordinates every activity in your body, including thought, speech, and language recognition; all your senses; and the functioning of your muscles and organs. Since many muscular problems as well as digestive, respiratory, and cardiovascular disorders have origins in the nervous system, a relaxed, healthy nervous system is essential for general health. Hence, the calming of the nervous system is a basic goal of Yoga therapy.

Functionally, there are two nervous systems that work side by side: the voluntary (VNS) and the autonomic nervous system (ANS).

The voluntary nervous system controls the functions of skeletal muscles—those that you move voluntarily. Nerves known as motor neurons carry messages from the brain to the muscles, allowing you to move your body the way you want.

The autonomic nervous system is not within your typical voluntary control. It directs involuntary functions such as those in the cardiovascular, respiratory, and digestive systems. The ANS controls your heart rate and whether your blood vessels are dilated or constricted (open or narrowed)—an important factor in migraines. Within the ANS, there are two complementary systems: the sympathetic and the parasympathetic nervous systems.

When the sympathetic nervous system is stimulated, you feel more alert and energetic; your heart rate accelerates, you breathe faster, and your muscles tense up. This system is responsible for the fight-or-flight response. The parasympathetic nervous system encourages the body to relax. It lowers the heart rate, slows the breathing, enhances muscle relaxation, and boosts digestion. Ideally, the sympathetic and parasympathetic nervous systems work together in a harmonious give and take to regulate your responses. One reason we practice Yoga breathing is to stimulate the parasympathetic nervous system, calming the muscles and all bodily functions.

Neurons and neurotransmitters are the essential components of the nervous system and are involved in headaches, particularly migraines. Neurons are cells that transmit signals within the nervous system, although they don't do this by direct contact with each other. An electrical impulse travels down the neuron, causing the neuron to release a chemical that passes a signal on to the next neuron. The chemicals are neurotransmitters, which have names you might recognize, such as serotonin and norepinephrine.

There are pain sensors in your skin and other organs throughout your body. When the pain sensors are stimulated, they send messages to the brain, where the pain signals are processed and you feel pain. When you are feeling emotionally healthy, some of the pain signals are decreased and you actually feel less pain. When you are under stress, the pain signals can pass all the way to the brain without being diminished, so the pain is worse. Therefore your emotional state and stress level have a direct influence on the degree of pain you feel in your body.

NERVOUS SYSTEM AILMENTS

The two most common types of headaches are tension headaches and migraines. Each can last from a couple of hours to several days, and the pain can be mild to severe. They can occur in both children and adults. Although they are unpleasant and can even be unbearable, these headaches are not in themselves dangerous. They do not cause any permanent damage, and do not stem from any other underlying medical condition, so they are called "primary headaches." There is a third type of primary headache called cluster headaches, but these only occur in about 1 percent of the population, usually in males. Cluster headaches come in groups over a few weeks, with excruciating pain, but then may disappear for months or years. Cluster headaches are similar to migraines, in that the blood vessels are involved.

While not all headaches require medical attention, if you have chronic or severe head pain you should see a doctor before starting Yoga or any other treatment. Although rare, it is possible to have "secondary headaches" that result from another condition and can be potentially fatal if untreated. Some of the most dangerous headaches are caused by brain tumors, ruptured aneurysms, and meningitis. However, an occasional mild headache during a stressful time or a mild upper respiratory infection is probably not harmful and does not necessarily require a visit to the doctor.

Tension Headaches

The mechanism for tension headaches is complex and includes problems with neurotransmitters within the brain, as well as aggravating factors such as external stress. Tension headaches are often described as a tight feeling around the head, like a band circling the head and squeezing. They sometimes feel like a tight hat above the eyes or cause neck pain that goes to the base of the skull. These headaches are felt on both sides of the head simultaneously, and feel like a steady ache rather than a throb. The pain can be mild or severe to excruciating, but there are usually no associated symptoms such as nausea.

Tension headaches are not dangerous but can be distressing or even debilitating. They often occur near the end of a stressful day, although some unlucky folks can wake up with a tension headache in the morning. The good news is that the practice of Yoga can be very successful in preventing and treating these headaches.

Migraines

The word *migraine* is French for the Greek *hemicranios,* meaning "half a head," because it typically occurs on only one side of the head.[2] The pain is usually described as throbbing or pounding, and it is frequently accompanied by nausea and vomiting. People with migraines usually feel the need to avoid bright lights and loud sounds, and would like to be able to sleep off the headache. About 10 percent of migraine sufferers get an "aura" before the headache begins, which may consist of flashing lights or other changes in vision. This aura can serve as a warning signal and an impetus to take the proper medication or begin an appropriate Yoga program immediately, to head off the migraine.

Migraine headaches are in the category of vascular headaches, meaning blood vessels are involved. Doctors once believed that migraines occurred when the blood vessels became constricted, leading to an aura, and then became dilated, leading to the head pain. It is now recognized that migraines may be related to a deficiency of neurotransmitters such as serotonin, but science is still lacking a complete understanding of their origins. Up to 90 percent of people with migraines have at least one family member who also has migraines.

Treatment for Headaches

If you are trying to get rid of your headaches, it is important to understand that there are a wide variety of treatments, and individuals respond differently to each of them. What works for one person may not work for another, and even for the same person, what works one time may not work the next. For this reason, the Yoga philosophy of treatment is to take a multifaceted approach to discover what might help.

There are quite a few different prescription and over-the-counter medications for headaches. One of the problems with treating frequent headaches with medication is the development of rebound headaches. Rebound headaches occur when the medicine used to treat the headache wears off and the pain reappears, often leading the sufferer to take more medicine. This is a difficult and painful catch-22 situation, because the best treatment for rebound headaches is to stop the medicine that seems so badly needed. Because of the phenomenon of rebound headaches, most doctors agree that frequent tension and migraine headaches are much better treated preventatively whenever possible, through medicines or other techniques such as Yoga.

Antidepressants may be used to prevent chronic headaches and frequent migraines. The antidepressants work by making more neurotransmitters available to transmit nerve signals. Some medicines that are used to treat high blood pressure (a vascular condition) can be used to prevent migraines.

The Yoga Advantage for Nervous System Ailments

Tara was in her late forties and had suffered from severe migraines for more than twenty years. She had seen numerous medical specialists and tried medications with limited success. For a year, her pain had been increasing to the point that she was requesting Demerol shots from her doctor. Since long-term migraines are a complex problem, I suggested we take a holistic look at her health and that we approach her migraines from several directions.

First I referred her to a physician who discovered that Tara's migraines were brought on by certain foods. This was a major breakthrough. Tara and her husband had joined a wine and cheese club just before the attacks had started escalating, but she had never made the connection until her physician suggested that she see what would happen if she eliminated wine and cheese from her diet. This initial step began to help. The next breakthrough was when I learned that Tara was a night owl, going to bed after midnight and getting up by 6:30 A.M. to get the kids off to school. One of the major tenets of healing headaches from a Yoga standpoint is to go to bed early and get plenty of sleep. Tara felt that getting to bed by 10:00 P.M. would be quite a challenge, but she agreed to give it her best shot.

I recommended Core Routine II (page 78) for Tara when she did not have migraine symptoms. I gave her a separate routine to practice when she first felt a headache coming on. This routine is outlined later in this chapter.

Tara practiced her Yoga on a daily basis and was pretty consistent with her diet and sleep improvements. After only a month, she noticed a significant decrease in headaches, and after two months Tara's symptoms had been reduced by half and she was no longer requesting Demerol injections. After a year and a half, Tara is almost headache free and elated with the new freedom this gives her. "I had to make some difficult changes," she told me, "and I wasn't sure I'd be able to do it. But being free of those migraines has given me a new lease on life, and that makes all the little sacrifices worthwhile."

Tara's situation perfectly illustrates the intricate nature of headaches, and the multifaceted approach that often is necessary to treat them. This can be true of all primary headaches, because they may have a variety of interrelated causes. Typical triggers of chronic headaches include food sensitivities, hormonal changes as in the menstrual cycle, inadequate sleep, change of weather, and emotional factors such as stress.

The primary use of Yoga for headaches is prevention. The Yoga philosophy helps headaches because it encourages you to look at yourself holistically and to consider all possible contributors to your headaches. If you are serious about eliminating your headaches, you may need to make some lifestyle changes.

The first step is to discover what sets off your headaches. If you have chronic headaches and haven't identified your personal triggers, you can benefit from keeping a diary in which you keep track of your headaches, noting their severity and any possible contributing factors that preceded the headache. Foods that commonly activate migraines are alcohol, aged cheeses, red wine, chocolate, dairy products, nitrates in hot dogs and lunchmeats, MSG, aspartame (NutraSweet), and changes in your usual amount of caffeine intake (either too much or too little). Environmental factors include perfumes and weather changes. You should also keep track of other possible contributors such as stress levels, amount of sleep, irregular eating patterns, hormonal changes, and any other medications you may be taking (see the Resource Guide).

One of the biggest contributors to both migraines and tension headaches is stress. Contrary to popular myth, the fact that stress plays a role in migraine doesn't mean it is a psychological disorder. Stress has the same effect on migraines as it does on other disorders such as asthma and heart disease: It doesn't cause them, but it can make them worse. Yoga is one of the best methods of stress reduction. Practicing Yoga can help relax the tight and contracted muscles that are involved in tension headaches. By preventing stress or minimizing the body's response to stress, Yoga can prevent the onset of a tension headache or migraine. According to Dr. Dean Ornish of the Preventative Medicine Research Institute, "Many people find that meditation and Yoga may help decrease the frequency of migraines, since stress may cause your arteries to constrict and stress management techniques may help to prevent this from happening in the first place."[3]

Yoga provides an effective alternative to medications because it doesn't lead to rebound headaches. For this reason, Dr. Richard Usatine works with his patients to approach their headaches holistically rather than simply prescribing medication. In more severe tension and migraines headaches, Yoga can be used safely in conjunction with medications.

Practicing a Yoga routine has specific benefits for headache sufferers in addition to general stress reduction. It can loosen up chronically tense muscles in the head, neck, and back. It can provide relief from sensory overload, and relax your mind so that your body can effectively combat pain. The Yoga philosophy overall can stop you from being locked in the viscous circle of pain-anxiety-more pain that leads to chronic headache problems.[4]

The Yoga Prescription for
Nervous System Ailments

※ Identify your dietary triggers and make a point to avoid them. You may want to start by steering clear of red wine, aged cheeses, chocolate, nitrates, and MSG.

※ Keep a headache diary to help discover your triggers.

※ Eat a healthy diet that's relatively low in fat and high in complex carbohydrates.

※ Sleep at least seven or eight hours per night. If you are doing this, and it doesn't seem to be working, try going to bed earlier and getting up earlier.

※ Try to isolate other environmental and lifestyle factors that bring on your headaches, and take steps to minimize or avoid them.

※ For long-term and severe pain, consult with your doctor to construct a multifaceted plan of attack, including medication if prescribed, avoidance of triggers, and daily Yoga practice.

※ Practice the appropriate Yoga therapy routine from this chapter. Start with two or three days a week, working up to five or six days a week.

YOGA FOR NERVOUS SYSTEM AILMENTS

Yoga for Migraines

For Prevention of Migraines: Use Core Routine II (page 78) once per day. Use Focused Breathing Part Two (page 39). Inhale and exhale through your nose, pausing briefly after the inhalation and the exhalation.

If Core Routine II is too difficult, practice Core Routine I (page 62) or the easier Lower Back Routine (page 114) for about two to four weeks each, and work up to Core Routine II.

At the First Sign of Migraine Symptoms: When you think a migraine is coming on, practice the Yoga Routine for Tension Headaches, as long as you feel you can.

During a Migraine: Do not practice Yoga during an acute migraine attack.

Yoga for Tension Headaches

One useful headache remedy is an ancient Yoga technique called the Six-Opening Seal. Traditionally, you would use your hands to partially seal off your eyes, ears, and nostrils. Yoga master B. K. S. Iyengar has popularized a modern adaptation using an elastic (Ace) bandage to wrap your forehead, ears, and eyes. This creates pressure and reduces sensory input to calm tension in the eyes and brain.

The following routine ends with three postures that call for the optional use of an elastic bandage. If you prefer not to use the bandage, just skip over it. This routine takes approximately fifteen to twenty minutes and should be practiced twice a day, once at the time you normally get your headaches, and one other time. Use Belly Breathing (page 41). Ideally, practice the routine twice a day until your condition improves, then practice it once a day. When you feel your condition has subsided, you may cut down to three times a week.

It is not dangerous to practice this routine when a tension headache is already present, and it can help alleviate the headache. However, it is best to start the routine before the onset of the headache.

Seated Posture

This posture is used for all seated positions in this routine. It supports the spine and facilitates a good sitting position.

1. Sit comfortably in an armless chair, bringing your body slightly away from the back rest.
2. Let your arms hang down by your sides. Place your feet evenly on the floor at hip width. If your feet do not touch the floor, place a folded blanket or a phone book under them. Your thighs should be parallel to the floor, with your knees and hips bent at approximately a 90 degree angle.
3. Place your hands on your thighs with your fingers toward your knees. Bring your back up nice and tall, and gently pull your head back until your ears, shoulder, and hip sockets are in alignment. Do not force anything beyond your comfort level.
4. Use Belly Breathing, for 8 to 10 breaths. Gently draw the belly in toward your spine on the exhale.

Seated Alternate Arm Raise

This movement improves range of motion and brings circulation to your upper back and shoulders.

1. Start in the Seated Posture.
2. Let your arms hang at your sides, palms turned back. Look straight ahead.
3. As you inhale, raise your right arm forward and up overhead until it is vertical.
4. As you exhale, bring your right arm down to the starting position.
5. As you inhale, raise the left arm forward and up overhead. Exhale on the return.
6. Repeat 4 to 6 times, alternating arms.

The Newspaper

This sequence relieves tension and promotes circulation in your upper back, neck, and shoulders.

1. Start in the Seated Posture.
2. Place your hands on your thighs, palms up. As you exhale, raise both hands to eye level, palms facing you as though you were holding an open newspaper.
3. As you inhale, move your open hands forward, up, and overhead. Follow your hands with your eyes and head. Stop when your hands are directly over your forehead.
4. As you exhale, bring only your chin down toward your chest.
5. As you inhale, bring your elbows back and apart from each other, turning your palms forward and flexing your wrists backward. Lift your chin off your chest and look straight ahead, pressing your elbows back.
6. As you exhale, round your back forward like a camel, bringing your bent arms forward so they are in front of you. Keep a slight bend in your elbows. Your arms should be roughly parallel to the floor, with your arms and ears in alignment.
7. As you inhale, return to the starting position; then fully exhale.
8. Repeat slowly 4 to 6 times.

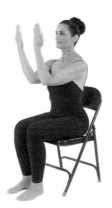
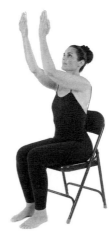

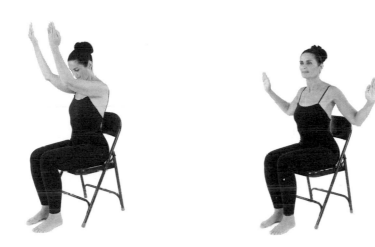

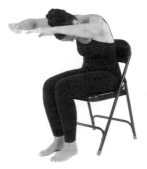

Seated Chair Twist

This gentle twisting motion stretches the muscles of your upper and lower back and tones the abdomen.

1. Sit sideways on a chair with the seat back to your right, feet flat on the floor and heels directly below the knees.
2. Exhale, turn to your right, and hold the sides of the chair back with your hands. If your feet are not comfortably on the floor, place a folded blanket or a phone book under them.
3. As you inhale, bring your back up tall, as if you were trying to touch the ceiling with the top of your spine.
4. As you exhale, twist your torso and head farther to the right.
5. Return to the starting position. Repeat the twist, gradually twisting farther with each exhalation for 3 breaths, but do not go beyond your comfort zone. On the last repetition, hold the twist for 6 to 8 breaths; then return to the starting position.
6. Repeat the same sequence on the opposite side.

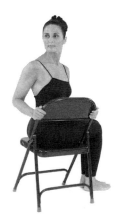

Sitting Cat

This posture relaxes and gently stretches your lower and upper back. (If you have knee or hip problems, replace Sitting Cat with Knees to Chest, described on page 200.)

1. Start on your hands and knees, looking slightly down, with the heels of your hands directly below your shoulders and your knees at hip width.
2. As you exhale, sit back on your heels and bring your head toward the floor. Work toward resting your torso on your thighs with your forehead on the floor, but do not force it. Sit back only as far as comfortable.
3. Repeat 3 times, and then relax with your head down and your arms in front (as in Step 2), for 6 to 8 breaths.

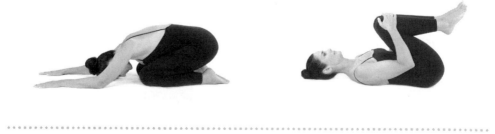

Apply the Elastic Bandage

If you'd like, an elastic (Ace) bandage can be used for the remaining postures. To apply it, start with the bandage rolled up. Hold the roll in your right hand, and with your left hand, press the free end against the back of your head. Start to wrap the bandage around your head. First wrap your forehead, then your ears and eyes, but not your nostrils. Wrap firmly, but not too tightly. If you wear contact lenses, it is best to take them out. When you are finished wrapping, slip the free end of the bandage under one of the folds.

If you do not want to wrap your eyes, just wrap your forehead. If your eyes are wrapped, simply slip the bandage up a little each time you need to see, then slip it back down again to cover your eyes in the pose.

Seated Forward Bend (Supported), Optional Elastic Bandage

This posture facilitates a general calming effect. It stretches the entire back of the body, including the neck, reducing symptoms of headache.

Caution: Be careful of seated forward bends if you have intervertebral disk problems. Check with your health-care professional if you are uncertain.

1. Sit on the floor, with your legs extended in front of you at hip width. Place a bolster under your knees and a pillow or blanket on your thighs.
2. Stretch your arms, hands, chest, and head over your thighs, and place your hands on your shins, ankles, or toes. Bending from the base of your spine, bring your waist, chest, and head forward; then relax.
3. Stay in this supported position for 2 to 5 minutes. If this posture feels uncomfortable, try it without the bolsters, blankets, or pillows.

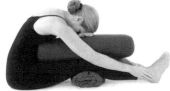

Corpse (Supported) with Two-Step Exhalation, Optional Elastic Bandage

If you are not comfortable in the supported Corpse, just lie flat on your back in the classic Corpse (page 70).

1. Lie on your back supported by pillows or folded blankets under your upper back, with your hips on the floor, your arms relaxed near your sides, and palms turned up. If your head or neck is uncomfortable, place a small pillow under it. If your lower back is uncomfortable, place a pillow under your knees or lower the support under your upper back.
2. Inhale fully. Draw in the belly as you exhale half of your breath in 3 to 5 seconds; then hold the breath for 3 to 5 seconds. Finally exhale the rest of your breath. If you find yourself gasping for air, shorten the length that you hold the breath, or use Belly Breathing (page 41) with a long exhalation.
3. Repeat 8 to 12 times.

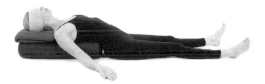

Relaxation Technique, Optional Elastic Bandage

1. Remain in the supported Corpse. Return to Belly Breathing (page 41).
2. Use Healing Triangles (page 52), Yoga Nidra (page 53), or Open-Ended Meditation (page 58), for at least 5 minutes.

Breathing Break

For general stress relief, take a breathing break once a day for three to five minutes, five to seven days a week. Use Alternate Nostril Breathing (page 45) or Victorious Breath (page 44).

12

For Women Only:

Menstrual Cramps, PMS, Menopause

As girls enter their teen years, they can hardly wait for the signs of womanhood to transform their bodies. They anticipate their new curves and monthly period, knowing these changes signify maturity and a profound change in their physical being. But often these new developments, once so welcome, begin to cause physical and emotional distress that can continue throughout a woman's adult life, culminating in another momentous bodily change—menopause—that has a reputation for causing a whole new form of suffering. Where did that old catchphrase "the joys of womanhood" come from, anyway?

Monthly menstrual cramps, premenstrual syndrome (PMS), and troublesome menopause have come to be accepted as normal aspects of a woman's life in the Western world. For generations, women have been told that their reproductive cycles and the changes that come with aging are mysterious syndromes, often causing pain, discomfort, and eventual loss of womanhood. In the Yoga view, these negative expectations are part of the problem. The Yoga philosophy encourages women to experience true integration of mind, body, and spirit, cultivating a more positive body image and easing the stress associated with normal reproductive functions. Through a Yoga practice, women can gain a healthier view of their cycles and achieve a degree of control over their physical, emotional, and spiritual well-being.

PHYSIOLOGY 101

The Monthly Cycle

A few words about the menstrual cycle will help in understanding the female difficulties we'll be addressing later in this chapter. (This is a general overview that applies to healthy women whose reproductive systems are working properly.)

Approximately once a month, a surge in the hormones estrogen and progesterone causes the inner lining of the uterus (the endometrium) to build up in preparation for a possible pregnancy. An egg is released by one of the ovaries, and if a sperm does not fertilize it, the lining of the uterus is no longer needed. Estrogen and progesterone levels decline, and molecular compounds called prostaglandins are released, causing the muscles of the uterus to contract. This constricts blood supply to the endometrium, blocking the delivery of oxygen to the tissue, which causes the endometrium to break down and die. The uterine contractions then squeeze the old endometrial tissue through the cervix and out of the body through the vagina (the monthly period). It will be replaced by a new lining in the next month.

Women's reproductive cycles are governed by hormones, whose levels rise and fall in a cyclical pattern throughout the month. These hormone levels have side effects and are partly responsible for many of the negative symptoms women experience related to menstruation and menopause. As women near the age of about fifty, hormone production declines and the monthly cycle slows and eventually stops, meaning they will not have periods and are no longer capable of bearing children naturally.

MENSTRUAL CRAMPS

As a teenager, probably one of the most unpleasant aspects of coming of age is the onset of menstrual cramps along with your first period. (The medical term for menstrual cramps is *dysmenorrhea*.) These abdominal and pelvic pains, felt before and during menstruation, can range from mild to quite severe. The discomfort can feel like heaviness in the belly; pressure in the groin; or debilitating aches throughout the abdomen, pelvis, and lower back.

As you get older, your cramps will usually diminish, especially after a pregnancy. This is thought to be due to the fact that the uterine nerves degenerate with age and disappear late in pregnancy, with only a portion of these nerves regenerating after childbirth. Menstrual cramps are caused by uterine contractions. The pain is intensified when clots or larger pieces of tissue pass through the cervix, especially if your cervical canal is narrow.

Yogis have long believed, and studies have confirmed, that emotional stress can increase the discomfort of menstrual cramps. Doctors have also seen that lack of exercise and inadequate rest seem to make cramps worse. Since Yoga relieves stress, exercises the body, and can enhance the body's ability to rest, it can be one of the best treatments for menstrual cramps.

Most women are aware of what their "normal" cramps feel like. If you begin to experience significant changes in the severity, timing, or location of your menstrual cramps, consult your physician, since there are a number of underlying conditions that can contribute to the pain. For regular discomfort that is not caused by an underlying disorder, the most common remedy is an over-the-counter anti-inflammatory such as ibuprofen. For mild cramps, aspirin or acetaminophen may be sufficient. You can effectively combine these remedies with Yoga to provide tremendous relief from monthly menstrual pain. If you suffer from menstrual cramps, be sure to read Yoga for Menstrual Cramps and PMS on page 226.

PREMENSTRUAL SYNDROME

Women's experiences of PMS vary widely and in fact, the diverse symptoms that make up PMS have been recognized and classified as a distinct syndrome only since the 1980s. Dramatic fluctuations of estrogen and progesterone throughout the month can give rise to physical challenges including headaches, abdominal bloating, swollen breasts, acne, fatigue, insomnia, joint pain, and water retention. But the emotional roller coaster can be even harder to deal with. Overwhelming feelings of anger, depression, and self-loathing can make the most basic functioning problematical. A few women get so despondent from the monthly hormonal imbalance that they contemplate suicide.[1]

Studies have shown that a change in diet can help alleviate some PMS symptoms. Reducing sugar, caffeine, alcohol, tobacco, and processed foods can help calm feelings of irritability and increase energy levels. As with menstrual cramps, regular exercise and control of stress can go a long way toward easing the monthly misery. Doctors often recommend a program of muscle relaxation or deep breathing exercises to help lessen headaches, anxiety, or trouble falling asleep. A practice of Yoga that encompasses daily routines as well as meditation, Breathing Breaks, and attention to overall wellness is shown to provide maximum relief for even the most miserable PMS sufferers. If you suffer from PMS, be sure to read our Yoga Routine for Menstrual Cramps and PMS on page 226.

MENOPAUSE

Women survive menstruation and PMS only to confront a new hormonal challenge: menopause. Unlike a disease that needs to be cured or prevented, menopause is a natural part of aging. Yogis view menopause as a reason for celebration, a time of deepening wisdom and insight. Released from the pressure and responsibility of childbearing, women have more freedom to focus on themselves, pursue their passions, and develop their spiritual awareness. Unfortunately, the physical difficulties of menopause combined with our youth-oriented society have made it hard for some women to imagine the potential blessings of this later stage of life.[2]

Menopause is the medical term for the time when you stop having menstrual periods. Natural menopause occurs when your ovaries stop releasing eggs and the lining of the uterus no longer sheds every month. This process happens gradually with the estrogen and progesterone levels decreasing over as many as ten years. When it's been a year since your last period and you haven't been pregnant, you've gone through menopause. The date of your last period is considered the onset of menopause. In the United States, the average age of menopause is fifty-one, but some women go through menopause closer to sixty, and some in their forties. If you have your ovaries removed, often done at the same time as a hysterectomy, it is called surgical menopause. Chemotherapy can also accelerate the onset of menopause.

Some women float through menopause with no intense symptoms, while many others suffer from an unpleasant array of emotional and physical problems. Probably the best-known sign of menopause is the hot flash, caused by decreasing levels of estrogen, which plays a role in regulating body temperature. You could start getting hot flashes several years before your periods stop, and they can continue for up to ten years after menopause. A hot flash is exactly what it sounds like: out of the blue, you suddenly feel so hot that you are uncomfortable and begin to sweat. Hot flashes can last thirty seconds to five minutes, and if they happen when you're sleeping, they can cause night sweats.

Decreased estrogen also causes a number of other problems. Vaginal dryness is common, leading to painful sex and an increase in vaginal and urinary infections. There is also a decreased blood flow to the vagina, which inhibits sensation and can reduce orgasmic response. Studies have not confirmed the role of menopause in sexual desire. Some women lose desire while others say they gain, and some report no change at all.

Protection against heart disease and possibly Alzheimer's is the major reason doctors recommend hormone replacement therapy (HRT) for some women. HRT involves taking two types of hormones, estrogen and progestin (although women who have had hysterectomies do not need the progestin). Taking these hormones protects against osteoporosis and may protect against heart disease and Alzheimer's. These hormones also treat hot flashes and other negative symptoms of menopause. However, there are risks involved, including possible blood clots, gallbladder disease, and a small increased incidence of breast cancer. The decision to begin HRT is a very personal one between you and your doctor, and should be carefully considered in light of your own medical history and physical health.

Other possible physical symptoms of menopause include fatigue, hair changes, headaches, heart palpitations, and weight gain. Emotional symptoms can consist of stress, anxiety, depression, tearfulness, irritability, insomnia, lack of concentration, and forgetfulness. Luckily, most women do not have every possible symptom.

The Yoga Advantage
for Women

While in many cultures the attribute that sets women apart from men, the ability to bear children, is a cause for reverence and celebration, in our society it is rarely celebrated and sometimes viewed as a burden. The fact that many women focus for most of their lives on avoiding pregnancy makes this special capability seem more like a liability. Through physical, mental, and spiritual dimensions, Yoga can help bring back some of the innate strength and joy in being a woman.

Menstrual cramps, PMS, and menopause have all been shown to be made better with exercise. As a gentle exercise that strengthens the body and increases flexibility, Yoga releases endorphins, chemicals in your body that literally make you feel good. Higher levels of endorphins help your body maintain a state of wellness and promote physical and emotional healing. Some Yoga postures can help ease uterine cramps by gently helping blood clots release from the uterine wall, move through the cervix, and pass out through the vagina. Other poses can help alleviate backaches through easy stretching.

We cannot overestimate the role that stress plays in making menstrual and menopausal discomforts worse. Demanding jobs, family responsibilities, and unprecedented busyness have filled most women's lives with record levels of stress. The menstrual cycle itself is stressful when it disrupts normal activities and becomes just one more thing you have to worry about. The well-documented stress relieving effects of Yoga can bring almost instant relief from many negative physical and emotional symptoms. This is not to suggest that PMS, cramps, and menopausal suffering are psychosomatic; but research has shown how stress profoundly affects physical functioning and perception of pain. So if you practice Yoga for no other reason than to combat stress, you will see improvement.

But Yoga does so much more than allay stress. Yoga positions have been proven to promote circulation throughout the body. This can stimulate the endocrine system, which helps encourage a healthy, balanced release of hormones.[3] Since hormone fluctuations are partly responsible for all of the female difficulties we've been discussing, using Yoga to help your body regulate hormones is an effective preventative measure.

Yoga addresses the emotional challenges as well as the physical. When you practice Yoga, you learn to slow down your mind and begin to process negative emotions rather than let them fester. Yoga promotes awareness of your inner needs and allows you to deal with them positively. Through deep breathing, stretching, and releasing bodily tension, your parasympathetic nervous system is stimulated, relaxing you and producing greater feelings of well-being. Most people emerge from a Yoga session refreshed and invigorated, without a trace of that nasty mood that might have plagued them before they started. Practicing Yoga regularly can help you control those volatile emotions and hang on to your good moods throughout the day no matter where you are in your cycle.

Women entering menopause often suffer from dwindling self-esteem related to getting older. Yoga provides positive reinforcement of the aging process by building self-awareness, increasing your energy and stamina, and improving posture, weight, and muscle tone so you can feel better about how you look.

According to Yoga wisdom, the time of the month when you are menstruating is a time of heightened awareness, when your natural insight and intuition become more prominent. This is also thought to be true during menopause. Your senses may be sharpened and you become more attuned to smells, sounds, textures, and tastes. Rather than let this increased sensitivity become a source of annoyance, you can use it to help you focus on the miraculous changes your body is experiencing and the positive aspects of simply being alive. From a spiritual perspective, these are times when meditation may be most powerful, freeing your mind from distractions and connecting you with a greater source of power, both within yourself and without. Yoga and meditation can be a natural doorway to the spiritual dimension and a means of transforming a troublesome time into a journey of self-discovery and joy.

The Yoga Prescription

for Women

❋ Engage in brisk walking, swimming, or other aerobic activity for twenty to thirty minutes at least three times a week to improve your overall health and fitness.

- Eat smaller, more frequent meals and limit salt to reduce bloating and fluid retention.
- Reduce or eliminate caffeine to lessen irritability, tension, and breast soreness.
- Avoid alcohol before your period or during menopause to minimize mood swings and depression.
- Eat a generally healthy diet, choosing foods high in complex carbohydrates (fruits, vegetables, and whole grains).
- Keep a journal of what you eat for a couple of weeks, to learn which foods seem to affect you negatively or exacerbate your symptoms.
- Make it a habit to get plenty of rest. Breathing and meditation techniques just before retiring can help you achieve more restful sleep.
- If you are particularly troubled by mood swings, try becoming more aware of your feelings throughout the day so you can use a breathing or relaxation technique when you need to stabilize your emotions or need to concentrate on a task.
- For hot flashes, try dressing in layers so you can remove something to cool off quickly. Use sheets and clothing that allow your skin to breathe, and try having a cold drink at the beginning of a flash.
- For vaginal dryness, use ointments that you can buy without a prescription such as K-Y jelly or Replens.
- Consider integrating meditation into your regular schedule, particularly during your period or if you are menopausal.
- Practice the appropriate Yoga therapy routine from this chapter. Start with two or three days a week, working toward five or six days a week.

Yoga for Menstrual Cramps and PMS

Practice Core Routine I (page 62) and Core Routine II (page 78) for general conditioning throughout the month, when you have no PMS symptoms and are not menstruating. Use Focused Breathing (page 39).

It is important not to strain or compress the abdominal area and to avoid inverted postures during your period, but aside from that you should not abandon your practice. The following is a routine I created for a client who suffered from PMS and painful cramps. Use it instead of the Core Routines when you have PMS symptoms or are having your period. This routine takes approximately twenty minutes and can be practiced up to three times per day, using Belly Breathing (page 41) with long exhalation.

Thunderbolt

You can use this posture as part of the routine, or by itself if you are having menstrual cramps or back pain. It is a relaxing pose that brings relief by promoting circulation in the abdomen. Do not do the Thunderbolt if you have knee problems.

1. Kneel on the floor or on a padded surface, knees and feet at hip width.
2. Sit back on your heels, and place your hands on the tops of your knees, elbows bent, palms down. Bring your back up nice and tall, and look straight ahead. If you are uncomfortable, you can place a pillow on your calves, so that when you sit down, it is between your calves and your buttocks. Increase the lift until you can sit comfortably. If you feel pain or tightness in the fronts of your ankles, place a rolled-up towel or blanket underneath them.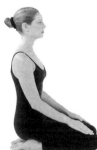
3. Start with 2 to 3 minutes, working up to 5 to 10 minutes.

Sitting Cat with Sound

This is a very nurturing posture that relaxes and gently stretches the back. The use of sound helps calm and relax the belly. (If you have knee or hip problems, replace Sitting Cat with Knees to Chest, described on page 229. Thus you will be doing Knees to Chest twice in this routine.)

1. Start on your hands and knees, looking forward and down, with the heels of your hands directly below your shoulders and your knees at hip width.
2. As you exhale, sit back slowly on your heels and bring your head toward the floor using the sound *ma* as you sit back. Work toward resting your torso on your thighs with your forehead on the floor, but do not force it. Sit back only as far as comfortable.
3. Move back to the starting position, then repeat Steps 1 and 2, alternating the sounds *ma* and *sa* for a total of 6 to 8 times.

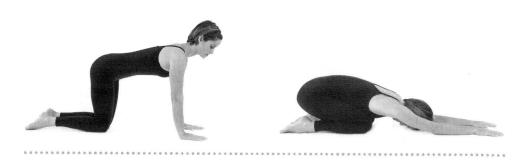

Reclined Bound Angle (Supported)

This relaxing posture loosens your hips and relaxes your lower back. It also promotes circulation in your pelvis.

1. Sit on the floor with your legs extended in front of you.
2. Lie back on a bolster, pillows, or folded blankets with your head supported by an additional blanket or pillow. Keep your hips on the floor.
3. Join the soles of your feet together with the bottom edge of both feet on the floor. Spread your knees wide and support them with bolsters or rolled blankets. Place your hands comfortably out to your sides, on the floor with your palms up. Cover your eyes with a towel or eye bag if you like.

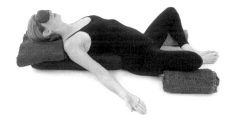

4. Stay in this position for 3 to 5 minutes. When you are ready to come out, place the soles of your feet on the floor, bring your knees together, and roll to one side.

Bridge

This is a good preparation for the supported Half Shoulder Stand that comes next. It promotes circulation in your back and neck, while strengthening your shoulders, hips, and thighs.

1. Lie on your back, bend your knees, and place your feet on the floor at hip width.
2. Relax your arms at your sides, palms down.

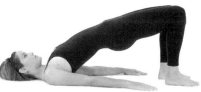

3. As you inhale, use your abdominal muscles to raise your hips halfway up. Pause. Then lift your hips as high as you feel comfortable. Do not go past halfway if it causes you any back pain.
4. As you exhale, bring your hips back to the floor.
5. Repeat 6 to 8 times, remembering to pause halfway up.

Half Shoulder Stand (Supported)

This inverted posture helps calm your nervous system and relaxes your lower back.

Caution: Do not use this or any inverted posture once menstruation has started.

1. Place a bolster or several folded blankets parallel to and about 6 inches away from a wall.
2. Sit sideways on the support, and then swing your legs up the wall. Rest the back of your pelvis on the support, and rest your head, neck, and shoulders on the floor.
3. Move your buttocks toward the wall until your sit bones are relaxed in the space between support and the wall. If you like, you may cover your eyes with a towel or eye bag.
4. Remain in this position for 3 to 5 minutes. When you are ready to come down, bring your knees toward your chest and slowly roll to one side.

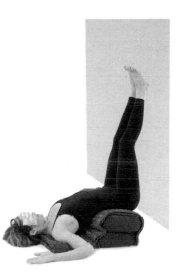

Knees to Chest

This soothing stretch relieves stiffness and discomfort in your lower back. It is great for releasing abdominal gas and for calming menstrual cramps. (Note that Knees to Chest is different from Knee to Chest, which appears elsewhere in the book.)

1. Lie on your back with your knees bent, feet on the floor at hip width. Bring your bent knees toward your chest and hold on to the top of your shins, just below your knees, one hand on each knee. If you are having knee problems, hold the backs of your thighs, under your knees.
2. As you exhale, draw your knees toward your chest. As you inhale, move your knees a few inches away from your chest, rolling your hips to the floor.
3. Repeat 6 to 8 times.

Cooling Breath

This breathing exercise calms and quiets your nervous system. It is described in detail on page 47. Sit in a comfortable position with your back up nice and straight. Slowly inhale and exhale. (If your tongue does not curl, do the Crow's Beak, described on page 47.) Repeat 8 to 12 times.

Corpse with Blankets

This is the safest and most popular Yoga posture, a classic for relaxation of the body and mind. It soothes the nervous system and facilitates deep rest.

1. Lie on your back with your arms relaxed near your sides and palms turned up. Place a bolster, pillows, or folded blankets under your upper back. If your head tilts back or your neck is uncomfortable, place a small pillow or blanket under your head and neck. If your lower back is uncomfortable, place a pillow or rolled blanket under your knees. If the supported position doesn't feel right to you, lie flat on your back in the classic Corpse.
2. Cover your eyes with an eye bag or folded towel.
3. Use the Healing Triangles (page 52) or Yoga Nidra (page 53) relaxation technique. Stay in the position for 5 to 15 minutes.

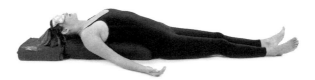

Breathing Break

Once per day, practice Alternate Nostril Breathing (page 45) for three to five minutes, and Focused Breathing Part Two (page 39) for an additional three to five minutes.

Yoga for Menopause

Practice Core Routine I (page 62) and Core Routine II (page 78) for general conditioning during menopause. You can alternate them if you like. Use Belly-to-Chest Breathing (page 41) or Chest-to-Belly Breathing (page 42).

Breathing Break

Once per day during menopause, practice Alternate Nostril Breathing (page 45) for three to ten minutes.

Meditation

It is a good idea to integrate meditation into your daily routine. Start slowly, aiming for about five minutes a couple of times a week. Gradually as you feel comfortable, work up to twenty to thirty minutes, five to seven days a week. Use any of the meditation techniques described in Chapter 5.

You may want to incorporate a mantra or affirmation into your meditation, especially if you're suffering from depression or low self-esteem. This is a positive statement to help reprogram your self-image. You can choose your own affirmation or use this one from the American Yoga Association: "I bless my body and accept its changes with grace and appreciation." Repeat your affirmation as you begin meditation, to help you focus. You can also repeat your affirmation upon rising in the morning and retiring at night, before meals, and whenever you start to have negative thoughts throughout the day.

13

Mental Health:

Anxiety and Depression

Our mental health is crucial for our total health and enjoyment of life. But millions of us are plagued with anxiety and/or depression, at some point in our lifetimes. The roots of psychological ailments often are the result of genetics, childhood wounds, and adult stresses. These disorders often run in families, with genetic predispositions and difficulties in the environment also contributing. If you are suffering mentally or psychologically, we implore you to get help. You may decide to see a psychologist, social worker, psychiatrist, or nurse therapist for individual therapy, or join a support group. Yoga can be your next step on the road to healing, after getting yourself under the care of a mental-health professional.

Many psychotherapists are aware of the benefits of Yoga. They've seen first-hand how practicing Yoga can put their clients in touch with themselves at a deep level. In this chapter, we are not suggesting that Yoga should replace psychotherapy or medication but that it can support the process of healing, adding depth to your self-examination and hastening recovery.

There are dozens of psychiatric disorders we will not discuss here. Ailments such as schizophrenia, bipolar disorder, and obsessive-compulsive disorder are complex mental health conditions requiring the care of a physician. For these and other psychiatric disorders, a general practice of Yoga can be helpful after the condition has been brought under control with medication and/or psychotherapy.

There is a biochemical component to most psychological problems, including anxiety and depression, and medical science has developed effective medications for targeting these irregularities in the brain and nervous system. For conditions requiring long-term medication, Yoga can help minimize certain side effects like fatigue and weight gain.

ANXIETY

Anxiety is a term for what we commonly call worrying. There are different levels of anxiety, ranging from an appropriate situational response to a dysfunctional condition. Anxiety about getting on a plane after a succession of airline crashes is not a disorder but a natural reaction to the environment. Deciding to never fly again is taking that anxiety to a level where it can interfere with your life.

For generalized anxiety disorder to be diagnosed, you must have excessive worry for at least six months, along with other symptoms such as restlessness, fatigue, difficulty concentrating, irritability, or sleep disturbance.[1] Chronic anxiety puts your mind and body in a perpetual state of stress, which drains energy and takes a toll on your health. Anxiety worsens with lack of exercise, which causes muscle tension to build. Even a short Yoga routine practiced daily helps regulate breathing and relax the body, releasing tension and bringing the mind from restlessness to stillness.

Panic disorder is anxiety related and characterized by the dramatic occurrence of a panic attack. This is a brief period of intense fear or discomfort with symptoms that included a pounding heart, sweating, trembling, chest pain, dizziness, and fear of dying.[2] It can last anywhere from five to thirty minutes. Medication and cognitive-behavioral therapy are often needed to stop recurring panic attacks. However, once a panic attack starts, Yoga breathing can be very helpful to end it.

Post-traumatic stress disorder (PTSD) is also classified as an anxiety disorder because of the similarity of symptoms. It is primarily a reaction to a traumatic and threatening event that causes you to feel intense fear, helplessness, or horror. The disorder is characterized by persistently recalling or reliving the event, including the associated emotions.[3] While therapy is usually needed to overcome PTSD, Yoga can help diminish the daily anxiety associated with it.

People with untreated anxiety-related conditions are at risk for depression, suicide, and substance abuse, as well as numerous other difficulties in living full, functional lives. Anxiety disorders do not clear up overnight nor do they disappear on their own, any more than a heart condition or diabetes would. The usual treatment is a combination of cognitive-behavioral therapy and medication. When using Yoga as part of the treatment, a commitment to practicing consistently for several months or years is recommended, since relapse is common in anxiety. You may experience periods of anxiety that are not quite severe enough to fit into one of the diagnoses described above, yet cause you distress and make functioning difficult. We recommend that you seek professional help anytime that anxiety gets in the way of your regular functioning. Your physician or therapist will discuss whether medications are potentially valuable for you. In some situations, psychotherapy combined with a regular Yoga practice may be enough to relieve your anxiety. If your anxiety is under control and you are ready to start a Yoga program, be sure to read Yoga for Anxiety on page 247.

DEPRESSION

Few of us can get through life without feeling depressed once in a while. A broken relationship, the loss of a job, or the death of a loved one can cause sadness and emotional pain, but there is a difference between feeling sad (depressed) and major depression.

Major depression descends over you like a black cloud, often for no apparent reason. It deadens your ability to feel joy or hope. It can make you feel worthless, apathetic, and desperately sad. Your mind is convinced that this bleak outlook will never change, that things will always be terrible. You can't just snap out of it, as your friends and family would like, and it may last for weeks, months, or years.[4]

Depression takes away interest and pleasure for most of the day, nearly every day. It affects your appetite, your sleep, and your ability to concentrate.[5] It rarely goes away on its own. When it does seem to disappear, it may be in remission and could strike again if you don't get help.

For all the awfulness of this disorder, the most tragic aspect may be the low percentage of those afflicted who seek and receive adequate treatment. Some studies show that as few as 10 percent of people with depression are properly treated for it. Part of the blame may be due to our society, which tends to view depression as some sort of moral failure and "personal weakness" rather than a bona fide health issue.[6]

Milder forms of depression include dysthymic disorder (a chronic, long-lasting low-level depression) and subclinical depression (which manifests fewer depressive symptoms and allows fairly normal functioning but still has a destructive impact).

Like anxiety, depression has a number of interlocking causal factors encompassing genetics, family history, and life circumstances. In recent years, the role of neurotransmitters (chemicals in the brain) has become better understood, and very successful antidepressant medications have been developed. These medications can make a significant difference to the lives of people with major depression. Even those with milder conditions can benefit by using the medication to lift the depression enough to boost the effectiveness of psychotherapy and lifestyle changes.

Once you have started to receive treatment for your depression, then you may safely begin Yoga. If fatigue and lack of motivation are part of your depression, then you can begin Yoga in small, easy doses with breathing exercises and simple postures. This will often help lift the sluggishness and lethargy that comes from depression, so that you are energized to try more. Initiating a Yoga practice may be difficult, but will become progressively easier once started.[7]

Practicing Yoga can considerably improve your mental state. However, do not stop your antidepressant medicine just because you are doing Yoga and feeling better. If you are considering stopping your medicine, please discuss the pros and cons with your doctor. If your depression is under control and you are ready to start a Yoga program, read Yoga for Depression on page 238.

The Yoga Advantage for Mental Health

The primary use of Yoga for mental health issues is to supplement whatever course of treatment you and your doctor have chosen. Regardless of your diagnosis, self-examination is going to be an integral aspect of your recovery. When you gently encourage your body and mind to go beyond its previous limits, as in practicing more advanced postures or increasing your meditation time, you discover strengths inside yourself you might not have known existed. This newfound strength can empower you to make unprecedented changes in your life.

With Yoga and especially meditation, part of the goal is always to control your thoughts. As discussed earlier in this book, Yoga is by definition "mindful" and cannot be practiced properly while your head is buzzing with a thousand random thoughts. In the beginning, controlling your thoughts is one of the most challenging aspects of Yoga. But with successive practice, you learn to recognize negative or destructive thoughts and consciously to replace them with something more positive. As you may have already discovered, this "thought recognition and replacement" is also a fundamental aspect of cognitive-behavioral therapy, the most effective psychotherapeutic technique for depression and anxiety disorders. So in a very concrete way, becoming skilled in your Yoga practice can contribute to your recovery.

There is evidence suggesting that people who are more physically active have a lower incidence of anxiety and depression. A major study in 1978 found that exercise was as effective in lowering symptoms among depressed patients as therapy.[8] Exercise, particularly a mindful exercise like Yoga, gets you in touch with your physical abilities and gives you tangible proof of your achievement. If you are practicing Yoga while undergoing treatment for your disorder, you will begin to have an overall sense of your own power, seeing that your efforts are capable of producing change. This can be a major attitude shift, especially if you've been mired in feelings of hopelessness and helplessness.

Medical research confirms Yoga's effectiveness for anxiety and depression. In 2001, a study involving fifty-four young adults showed significant decrease in anxiety and depression during and after ten months of consistent Yoga practice.[9] A 1999 study showed that Yoga reduced general anxiety levels, lowered irritability, and increased subjects' optimistic outlook on life.[10] Even more encouraging, a 1995 study showed that anxiety patients who learned meditation as part of their treatment maintained the positive benefits for at least three years, showing that Yoga's benefits are not just for today but can be a long-term solution.[11]

The Yoga Prescription for
Mental Health

※ See a physician and/or mental-health professional and get your condition under control before doing anything else.

※ Enlist the support of a trusted friend or relative to encourage you on your path to healing. It will be most helpful if this person can also practice Yoga with you, when you are first starting out.

※ Eat a healthy diet. See a nutritionist or get help from one of the many good books available (see Resource Guide).

※ Reduce your intake of caffeinated coffee and tea.

※ Although your condition may adversely affect your sleep, do your best to get a consistent seven to eight hours of sleep each night. Rising at the same time each morning can help regulate your body clock and sleep pattern.

※ Practice Yoga breathing so that you are able to rely on it in acute circumstances when you may need it, such as an impending panic attack.

※ Learn to recognize your body's signals that anxiety is building up, such as increased heart rate, tense muscles, and repetitive negative thoughts. Use Yoga breathing techniques to reverse the cycle.

※ For anxiety you can benefit tremendously from a regular practice of meditation, following the guidelines in given Chapter 5. For depression, it is best to delay starting meditation until your depression has lifted to some extent and you've discussed it with your therapist.

※ If depression makes it difficult for you to begin exercise, start Yoga very slowly by spending a few minutes a day doing Yoga breathing exercises. You can do this for a week or more until you feel ready to begin a routine.

※ Commit to practicing Yoga for at least six months to a year. Recovering from anxiety or depression is a long-term process.

※ When you are ready, practice the appropriate Yoga therapy routine from this chapter. Start with two or three days a week, working toward five to six days a week.

Yoga for Depression

This classic routine is similar to the one I learned at a Yoga therapy seminar for mental health in Scotland. Over the years I have seen it help countless people of all ages suffering from depression, and it is a safe and effective general conditioning program as well. This routine takes approximately twenty to twenty-five minutes and should be practiced using Chest-to-Belly Breathing (page 42) or Focused Breathing (page 39). Ideally, practice the routine twice a day until your condition has subsided, then you may cut down to three times a week.

....

Mountain Posture

The Mountain Posture is the cornerstone for all standing postures, and you will be using it throughout this routine. It improves posture and spinal alignment, creating stability in your stance and facilitating breathing.

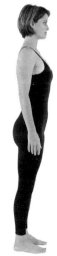

1. Stand with your feet at hip width. Keep your spine tall but relaxed. Let your arms hang at your sides, palms turned inward toward your legs.
2. Align the middle of your ear; your shoulder; and the sides of your hip, knee, and ankle along an imaginary vertical line.
3. Look straight ahead.
4. Remain in this posture for 8 to 10 breaths.

....

Rejuvenation Flow

This sequence stretches and strengthens the muscles of your trunk, arms, and legs, promoting circulation throughout your body.

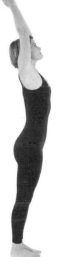

Caution: Be careful of forward bends if you have intervertebral disk problems. Check with your physician or healthcare professional if you are uncertain.

1. Start in the Mountain Posture.
2. As you inhale, raise your arms out to the sides, up, and overhead. Pause briefly.
3. Start your exhalation and bend forward from your hips, bringing your arms, hands, torso, and head forward toward the floor. Keep your arms and legs soft, and let your hands touch the floor or hang as close as they will go. Pause in this position.

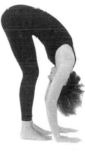

4. As you inhale, bend your knees deeply without lifting your heels off the floor, and sweep your arms out to the sides like wings. Arch your lower back like a saddle and bring your torso up until it is approximately parallel to the floor. Look at a point on the floor 3 feet in front of you. Pause briefly.
5. As you exhale, float down again and hang your arms to the floor as in Step 3.
6. As you inhale sweep your arms from the sides and bring your head and back all the way up to the standing position with arms overhead as in Step 2.

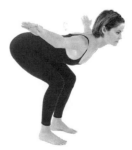

7. As you exhale, bring your arms back to your sides and return to the starting position.
8. Repeat the sequence 4 to 6 times. Remember to pause briefly after the inhale and the exhale.

Warrior I

This lunge-like posture strengthens your legs, back, shoulders, and arms. It helps improve stamina and balance and increases flexibility in your hips.

1. Start in the Mountain Posture. Take a big step forward with your right foot, approximately 3 feet for taller people, less if you are shorter. Your right knee should be directly over your ankle, and your thigh should be parallel to the floor. Place your hands on your hips and square your hips forward. Keep both legs straight and hang your arms at your sides in the ready position.
2. As you inhale, raise your arms forward and up overhead, and at the same time bend your right knee to a right angle. You should feel like you're in a classic runner's stretch, with a light pull in your left calf.
3. As you exhale, straighten your right leg and bring your arms back to the ready position as in Step 1.
4. Repeat 3 times, then hold Step 2 (Warrior I posture) for 6 to 8 breaths. Straighten up.
5. Repeat on the left side.

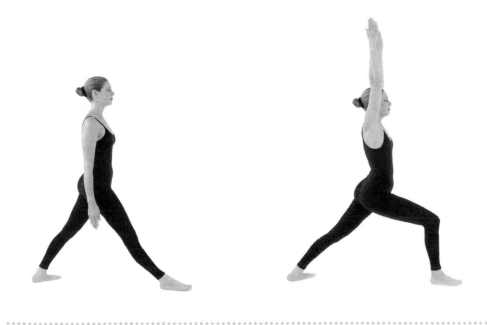

Revolved Triangle

This gentle twisting posture stimulates circulation to your spine, opens your hips, and stretches your hamstrings and calves. It also strengthens your neck, shoulders, and arms.

1. Start in the Mountain Posture. Step out to the right with your right foot in a wide stance, approximately 3 feet for taller people, less if you are shorter.
2. As you inhale, raise your arms out to the sides, parallel to the floor in a T.
3. Exhaling, bend forward from your hips, and then, in a twisting motion, place your right palm or fingers on the floor near the inside of your left foot. Continue exhaling. Raise your left arm into a vertical position and look up at your left hand. To make the posture easier, soften your left knee and arms, or move your right hand back to the right, below the midline of your torso. To make the posture more challenging, straighten your leg and place your right hand just outside of your left foot.
4. Repeat 3 times, and then hold Step 3 for 6 to 8 breaths.
5. Repeat the same sequence on the other side. Return to the Mountain Posture.

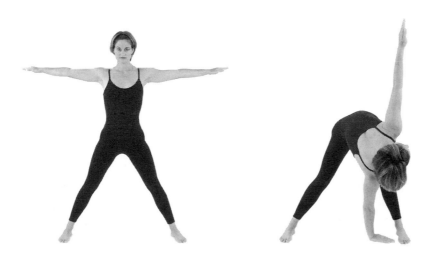

Standing Spread-Leg Forward Bend

This forward bend increases circulation to your upper torso and head. It opens your hips and stretches the backs and insides of your legs, including your hamstrings and adductors.

1. Start in the Mountain Posture. Step out to the right with your right foot in a wide stance, approximately 3 feet for taller people, less if you are shorter. As you inhale, raise your arms out from the sides forming a T with your torso.

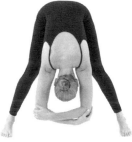

2. As you exhale, bend forward from the hips and hang down, holding each of your bent elbows with the opposite side hand. Soften your knees to where you are comfortable.
3. Stay in the folded position for 6 to 8 breaths.

Karate Kid

This balancing posture improves concentration, balance, and stability. It contributes to flexibility in your hips and strengthens your legs, arms, and shoulders.

1. Start in the Mountain Posture.
2. As you inhale, raise your arms out to the sides in a T, not higher than your shoulders.
3. Focus on a spot on the floor 6 to 8 feet in front of you. Exhaling, bend your right knee, lifting it toward your chest.
4. Hold for 6 to 8 breaths.
5. Repeat with your left knee.

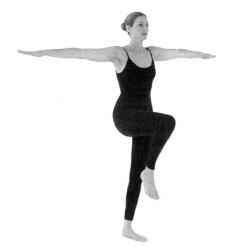

C o b r a

The Cobra increases the flexibility of the lower back and strengthens the arms, chest, and shoulders. It opens the chest, promoting a deeper breathing pattern.

Caution: If the Cobra causes any pain or discomfort, replace it with the Sphinx (described next). If both postures cause discomfort, leave them out.

1. Lie flat on your belly, legs at hip width, with the front of your feet on the floor. If you have lower back problems, it is important to separate your legs slightly wider than your hips and to turn your heels out.
2. Rest your forehead on the floor, and relax your shoulders. Place your palms on the floor with your thumbs near your armpits and your fingers facing forward. Your elbows should be bent close to your sides.
3. Inhaling, engage your back muscles, push your palms down against the floor, and lift your chest and head, looking straight ahead.
4. Leave the front of the pelvis on the floor, and keep your shoulders dropped and relaxed. Push yourself as high as feels comfortable, keeping your elbows bent unless your back is very flexible. To make this easier, move your hands farther forward. To make it more challenging, move your hands farther back.
5. Exhaling, lower your torso and head slowly back to the ground.
6. Repeat the lift 6 to 8 times.

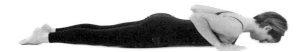

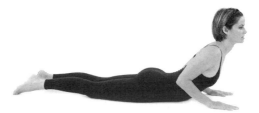

Sphinx (Substitute for the Cobra)

Use the Sphinx if you are not ready for the Cobra. The Sphinx emphasizes flexibility of the upper back and strengthens the arms, chest, and shoulders. It opens the chest, promoting a deeper breathing pattern.

1. Lie flat on your belly, legs at hip width, tops of your feet on the floor.
2. Relax your forehead on the floor, and release your shoulders. Place your forearms on the floor, palms turned down, near the sides of your head.
3. As you inhale, push your forearms against the floor, and lift your chest and head. Look forward and straight ahead. Your forearms and the front of your pelvis should stay on the floor. Try to keep your shoulders relaxed.
4. As you exhale, slowly lower yourself down to the floor.
5. Repeat the lift 6 to 8 times.

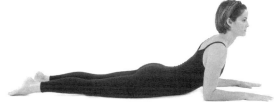

Sitting Cat

This posture relaxes and gently stretches the lower and upper back. We often use it to balance out the body after a bending posture. (If you have knee or hip problems, replace Sitting Cat with Knees to Chest, described next.)

1. Start on your hands and knees, looking forward, with the heels of your hands directly below the shoulders and the knees at hip width.
2. As you exhale, sit back on your heels and bring the head toward the floor. Work toward resting your torso on the thighs with your forehead on the floor, but do not force it. Sit back only as far as comfortable.
3. Repeat 3 times, and then relax with your head down and your arms in front (as in Step 2), for 6 to 8 breaths.

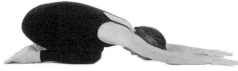

Knees to Chest (Substitute for Sitting Cat)

Do this posture only if you have hip or knee problems and cannot do Sitting Cat. The slow stretching motion relieves stiffness and discomfort in the lower back. (Note that Knees to Chest is different from Knee to Chest, which appears elsewhere in the book.)

1. Lie on your back with your knees bent, feet on the floor at hip width. Bring your bent knees toward your chest and hold on to the top of your shins just below your knees, one hand on each knee. If you are having knee problems, hold the back of your thighs under your knees.

2. As you exhale, draw your knees toward your chest. As you inhale, move your knees a few inches away from your chest, rolling your hips to the floor.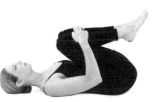

3. Repeat 3 times, and then stay in the most folded position for 6 to 8 breaths.

Shining Skull Breath

This is an invigorating breathing exercise, described in detail on page 46. Do it seated comfortably in a chair or on the floor, starting with 15 to 20 breaths. After a few days, you can increase your repetitions, doing 25 to 35 breaths.

Corpse with Blankets

This is the classic Yoga posture for relaxation of the body and mind. It soothes the nervous system and facilitates deep rest.

1. Lie on your back with your arms at your sides, palms up. Place pillows, blankets, or a bolster under your upper back to gently open the chest. Keep your hips on the floor and place blankets or pillows under your head and neck for support. If your back is uncomfortable, place a rolled blanket under your knees or lower the support under the upper back.
2. Close your eyes and relax. You may cover your eyes with a folded towel or eye bag if you like.
3. Use the Yoga Nidra (page 53) relaxation technique with the affirmation given below.
4. Relax for at least 5 minutes.

Affirmation

An affirmation is a positive statement or prayer, repeated verbally or mentally to help reprogram your subconscious mind. You can choose your own affirmation or use the following: "Every day, in every way, I grow stronger with my body, breath, and mind." Repeat your affirmation upon rising and on retiring at night, before meals, during your relaxation exercise (Yoga Nidra), and whenever you start to have negative thoughts throughout the day.

Breathing Break

For general stress relief, once per day practice the Shining Skull Breath (page 46) for two rounds of eight to twelve breaths, and Chest-to-Belly Breathing (page 42) for five minutes.

Yoga for Anxiety

Practice Core Routine II (page 78). If Core Routine II is too difficult, practice Core Routine I (page 62) or the easier Lower Back Routine (page 114) for about two to four weeks each and work up to Core Routine II. Practice using Focused Breathing (page 39) or Chest-to-Belly Breathing (page 42). Ideally, practice the routine twice a day until your condition improves, then practice it once a day. When you feel your condition has subsided, you may cut down to three times a week.

When you get to the end of the routine, replace the final Corpse posture and Relaxation Technique with the following two exercises.

Alternate Nostril Breathing

This breathing exercise creates balance and harmony. It is described in detail on page 45. Do it seated comfortably in a chair or on the floor. Repeat the cycle 8 to 12 times. In your first session practicing this technique, start with inhalations and exhalations of about five to seven seconds each. Over time as you continue to practice, gradually increase the length of your breath until you reach your comfortable maximum.

Corpse with Yoga Nidra

This is the classic posture for relaxation of the body and mind. It soothes the nervous system and facilitates deep rest.

1. Lie on your back with your arms at your sides, palms up. If your head tilts back or your neck is uncomfortable, place a small pillow under it. If your back is uncomfortable, place a rolled blanket under your knees. Close your eyes and relax.
2. Use the Yoga Nidra (page 53) relaxation technique with the affirmation on the next page.
3. Relax for at least 5 minutes.

Affirmation

You may want to compose your own affirmation that applies directly to your situation. Repeat your affirmation upon rising and on retiring at night; before all meals; and whenever you start to have negative thoughts or fears throughout the day.

Some people find comfort in reciting this portion of The Prayer of Saint Francis of Assisi.

> Lord, make me an instrument of your peace.
> Where there is hatred, let me sow love;
> where there is injury, pardon;
> where there is doubt, faith;
> where there is despair, hope;
> where there is darkness, light;
> and where there is sadness, joy.

Breathing Break

For general stress relief, once per day practice Alternate Nostril Breathing (page 45) and Victorious Breath (page 44) for 3 to 5 minutes each.

14

The Endocrine System:

Diabetes, Obesity

L ate in the year 2001, the U.S. Centers for Disease Control and Prevention (CDC) released a report that should have been front-page news. It was an alarming account of the dramatic and parallel rise in the incidence of both obesity and diabetes. Calling these two health concerns "twin epidemics," CDC Director Dr. Jeffrey P. Koplan warned, "If we continue on this course for the next decade, the public health implications in terms of both disease and health care costs are staggering."[1] Dr. Koplan called on the health-care industry, along with schools and communities, to intensify efforts to prevent and treat these epidemics. Maybe the most striking aspect of the report was the admission that both diabetes and obesity are largely preventable through proper diet and exercise, yet over 60 percent of Americans are overweight and about fifteen million of us have diabetes. This means that more than half of the population is affected, and many people will die prematurely owing to their own unhealthy lifestyles.

Diabetes is a disease of the endocrine system, the system in our bodies responsible for producing and distributing hormones. It is caused by a lack of insulin, a hormone produced by the pancreas, or the ineffective action of insulin in the body. In type 1 diabetes, the pancreas stops producing insulin and the person with this condition must take insulin daily to stay alive. In type 2 diabetes, the pancreas is still producing insulin but the body is resistant to the insulin and does not use it effectively. In both types of diabetes, the lack of insulin activity results in high blood sugars and all the complications of diabetes.

Persons with type 1 diabetes always need to take insulin. In addition, proper diet, exercise, and weight control are an important part of controlling the diabetes and preventing complications. The major complications of diabetes are eye disease, foot problems, heart disease, and kidney problems.

Type 2 diabetes can often be treated by proper diet, exercise, and weight control alone. When lifestyle changes don't work well enough to bring the blood sugar under control, oral medications are prescribed. Some persons with type 2 diabetes will need to take insulin when the oral medications are not working adequately. One of the biggest risk factors for type 2 diabetes is obesity, which is caused by a complex relationship of genetics and behavior. Obesity can be partially caused by endocrine system problems, such as incorrect levels of thyroid hormones, insulin, or sex hormones. For this reason, we are covering obesity here along with the endocrine system. Keep in mind that most people who are overweight do not have a problem with their endocrine system; but if their weight problem continues, it's possible they eventually *will* have an endocrine problem—diabetes.

PHYSIOLOGY 101

The Endocrine System

The endocrine system is made up of glands throughout the body that secrete hormones—chemical messengers that regulate bodily processes such as growth, metabolism, and sexual development. The endocrine system keeps our body in balance through the function of hormones. The master gland is the hypothalamus, a tiny cluster of brain cells that receives messages from the body and transmits signals to the pituitary gland. The pituitary gland makes hormones in answer to the body's needs. These pituitary hormones signal other endocrine organs, such as the adrenal gland, thyroid gland, ovaries, and testes, to produce the hormones needed for good health. The ovaries (in females) and testes (in males) receive the messages from the pituitary and in turn produce the sex hormones—estrogen and progesterone in women, testosterone in men.

The pancreas is another gland that affects digestion. It lies behind the stomach. This gland secretes digestive juices that break down fats, carbohydrates, proteins, and acids. Within the pancreas are specialized cells that secrete hormones—glucagon and insulin—that together regulate the level of glucose in the blood. If the pancreas fails to produce insulin or secretes it in low quantities, the result is diabetes.

ENDOCRINE SYSTEM AILMENTS

Diabetes

In diabetes, your body does not properly produce or use insulin, a hormone needed to convert sugar, starches, and other food into energy needed for daily life. Type 1, in which patients require daily insulin injections to stay alive, makes up only 5 to 10 percent of diabetes cases. Type 2 diabetes is much more common. It is type 2 diabetes that the CDC reports is nearing epidemic proportions, and doctors believe it is due to the rise in obesity, sedentary lifestyles, and unhealthy diets.[2]

Controlling your diet is crucial when you have diabetes. Lowering fats, sugar, and alcohol and eating healthy amounts of whole grains, vegetables, and protein are the general guidelines. The book *Diabetes Meal Planning Made Easy: How to Put the Food Pyramid to Work for Your Busy Lifestyle,* sanctioned by the American Diabetes Association, shows you how to create a nutritional plan that works (see Resource Guide).

Exercise is one of the best ways to improve your health if you are diabetic, helping you lose weight and normalize blood sugar. However, you need to be careful about your blood sugar during exercise. It helps to have eaten relatively recently before exercising and to test your blood before and after exercise, especially if you take insulin. Most important, exercise should be done regularly, several days a week.

If you have obesity and diabetes simultaneously, healthy weight loss through diet and exercise can cause type 2 diabetes to disappear entirely. If you are steadily losing weight and staying healthy, be sure to get tested regularly by your doctor. Your diabetic medications will probably be lowered and may eventually be completely discontinued. If you have type 2 diabetes, be sure to read Yoga for Type 2 Diabetes and Obesity on page 256.

Obesity

Being overweight is a disheartening predicament that over half of Americans find themselves in. Doctors now determine whether and how much a person is overweight by figuring his or her body mass index (BMI). This measure is the ratio of your height to your weight (see Appendix C). Percentage of body fat is another reliable indicator of whether or not you are at a healthy weight, and some experts believe it may be a more accurate gauge than BMI.[3] One advantage of BMI is that it's easy to figure on your own with the help of a calculator, whereas you may not be able to get an accurate body fat percentage without seeking professional help. The bottom line is that weight, body fat, and BMI are all good tools for helping you determine where you lie on the healthy-weight spectrum. You should use them to help in your self-evaluation, but also consider how you feel, how many illnesses you tend to get, your energy levels, and how you look in the mirror.

Obesity has immense health risks. Heart disease, high blood pressure, stroke, and diabetes vastly increase with obesity, and the musculoskeletal system can be affected, most commonly by lower back pain, knee pain, arthritis, and carpal tunnel syndrome.

The best way to approach obesity is through a threefold plan of attack: Get your diet under control, find the amount and types of exercise that work for you, and find strategies that can help you maintain your resolve. These may include stress management, nutritional counseling, keeping a journal of your eating and exercise patterns, psychotherapy, accountability to another person, and mind–body practices that can increase your self-awareness and sense of personal power. See the Resource Guide for some diet book recommendations. If you are seriously overweight, be sure to read Yoga for Type 2 Diabetes and Obesity on page 256.

The Yoga Advantage for
Endocrine Ailments

The key to controlling body weight and diabetes is lifestyle. We all need to develop the discipline to exercise regularly and choose healthy foods. One of the greatest benefits of Yoga is that it helps you develop self-control. As you practice Yoga, you become more skilled at concentrating, and you learn to manage your thought processes. This can increase your willpower to make changes, even if they are difficult or unpleasant, such as cutting back on sweets.

People are often waylaid from their best intentions for diet and exercise by stress. Once you have a regular and reliable means of controlling stress, you can count on more success with your self-discipline. As we've discussed throughout this book, Yoga is one of the most effective stress busters available. Yoga is also known for increasing general feelings of well-being. When you're happy and content, it is easier to make choices that contribute to your health rather than your momentary pleasure.

Controlling stress can also have very concrete benefits in controlling diabetes. A landmark study of people with diabetes released in 2002 showed that stress-management techniques, including relaxation and breathing exercises, can significantly reduce the average glucose level, the important factor in diabetes. The effect was so great that the researchers compared it to the change they would expect to see from some diabetes-control drugs, and they concluded that "Managing stress can significantly improve a patient's control of their diabetes."[4]

Yoga is an ideal form of exercise if you are overweight. It is gentle and doesn't push you beyond your limits. It can be successfully practiced even by overweight individuals who may have given up on exercise because it was too difficult. Yoga does not strain the heart and when carefully practiced, has a very low risk of injury.

For people with diabetes, Yoga is a healthy form of exercise because it does not burn calories and bring down blood sugars as rapidly as more vigorous exercise such as jogging or aerobics. Because Yoga is usually done indoors in places where there is access to food or drinks, it is more likely that you will have some food available for treatment if your blood sugar should drop drastically.

Lydia was 46 and had been healthy all her life, but at age 42 she went through a difficult divorce and a long bout of depression. She gave up exercise and gradually her diet deteriorated, leading her to put on weight. Eventually her doctor diagnosed type 2 diabetes and obesity, put her on medication, and advised her to improve her diet. Her symptoms improved but she still suffered from fatigue, depression, and irritability, so Lydia's physician referred her to me. I worked closely with Lydia on her diet, increasing whole grains, beans, and vegetables and reducing fats, sweets, and alcohol. For exercise, she began walking regularly and practicing a daily Yoga routine similar to the one in this chapter. Her symptoms improved after only two weeks, and after three months she had lost sixteen pounds and her glucose levels had significantly decreased, so her doctor cut her medication dose in half. Lydia may continue to need medication for her diabetes, but she is much healthier and reports feeling great.

Being overweight can take a major toll on our self-esteem, reminding us of our perceived failures and lack of ability to change. One of the greatest advantages of Yoga is that it helps you see yourself in a different way. You can leave behind your disappointing image of yourself to discover your inner strength and the ability to make real changes in your life. Yoga is a gentle way to bring a balanced attitude to all aspects of life. If you commit to a regular practice and embrace all the principles of Yoga as explained in this book, you can achieve permanent weight loss, decrease or eliminate symptoms of diabetes, and rebuild your self-esteem to embrace life with confidence.

The Yoga Prescription for Endocrine Ailments

- Be informed about diabetes and/or obesity by reading books and accessing reliable information on the World Wide Web.
- Do some type of moderate aerobic exercise for at least twenty minutes, three to four times per week. Depending on your fitness level, you may want to start with walking, swimming, or cycling. Find an exercise you truly enjoy to increase your chances of keeping it up.
- Create a diet plan that works for you, referring to reliable sources and experimenting until you feel you're in a good groove. Avoid fasting or extreme fad diets.

❋ Choose a diet with plenty of grain products, vegetables, and fruits and that's low in fats and sugars.

❋ Make it a habit to sit down while eating. Eat slowly, savoring each bite. Do not eat while distracted by television, crime-filled newspapers, or a stressful conversation.

❋ Maintain regular sleep habits, getting seven to eight hours each night, a crucial component in protecting your overall health.

❋ If your BMI is 30 or higher, be sure to seek medical care and be aware of any health issues you may be facing due to obesity.

❋ Keep a journal of your food intake and exercise for a couple of weeks, as a reality check. Use that information to determine what you might need to modify.

❋ Consider therapy or an accountability program in which you report periodically to a counselor or nutritionist to discuss your progress.

❋ Take proactive steps to reduce the stress in your life.

❋ Integrate meditation into your schedule, following the guidelines given in Chapter 5.

❋ Practice the appropriate Yoga therapy routine from this chapter. Start with two or three days a week, working toward five to six days a week.

For Diabetes

❋ Time your exercise according to your meals and insulin. Generally, you want to exercise one to two hours after a meal.

❋ Be prepared to treat low blood sugar. Always carry juice, nondiet soft drink, glucose gel, raisins, or another fast-acting source of sugar. If you feel a reaction coming on, stop, test, and treat it right away.

❋ Be careful of your feet when you exercise or practice Yoga. You should not exercise in bare feet (except in a pool) and should use socks and appropriate footwear.

❋ If you drink alcoholic beverages, have no more than a drink or two, a few times a week. Never drink to intoxication.

❋ Enlist the help of a registered dietitian who has experience working with people who have diabetes. To find a registered dietitian near you, contact the American Diabetes Association.

Yoga for Type 2 Diabetes and Obesity

This routine is similar to the one I created for Lydia. It takes about twenty minutes, and should be practiced using Belly Breathing (page 41) or Focused Breathing Part Two (page 39). Inhale and exhale through the nose slowly, with a slight pause after both the inhale and the exhale. Ideally, practice twice a day until you are within your healthy weight range or your diabetes is under control. Then you can practice once a day.

Seated Posture

This basic posture will used throughout the routine.

1. Sit comfortably in an armless chair, bringing your body slightly away from the back rest.
2. Let your arms hang down by your sides. Place your feet evenly on the floor at hip width. If your feet do not touch the floor, place a folded blanket or a phone book under them. Your thighs should be parallel to the floor with your knees and hips bent at approximately a 90 degree angle.
3. Place your hands on your thighs with your fingers toward your knees. Bring your back up nice and tall, and gently pull your head back until your ears, shoulders, and hip sockets are in alignment. Do not force anything beyond your comfort level.
4. Hold for 8 to 10 breaths.

Seated Alternate Arm Raise

This simple arm movement gently stretches the muscles of the upper and lower back. It also promotes circulation to your neck and shoulders.

1. Start in the Seated Posture.
2. Let your arms hang at your sides, palms turned back. Look straight ahead.
3. As you inhale, raise your right arm forward and up overhead until it is vertical.
4. As you exhale, bring your right arm down to the starting position.
5. As you inhale, raise your left arm forward and up overhead. Exhale on the return.
6. Repeat 4 to 6 times, alternating arms.

Wing and Prayer

This simple movement gently works your upper back and opens up your chest.

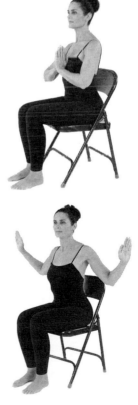

1. Start in the Seated Posture
2. As you exhale, join your palms in the prayer position, thumbs at the breastbone.
3. As you inhale, separate your hands and stretch your arms like wings to the sides at shoulder height. Your wrists stay flexed, your fingers pointing toward the ceiling and your palms facing away from you. Look straight ahead.
4. As you exhale, join the palms again at the breastbone.
5. Repeat 4 to 6 times.

Seated Chair Twist

This gentle twisting motion tones the abdomen and rejuvenates the spine.

Caution: Move carefully and slowly while executing a twist. If you experience any pain or discomfort, leave the twist out of your routine until you can check with your health-care professional.

1. Sit sideways on a chair with the chair back to your right, feet flat on the floor, and heels directly below your knees.
2. Exhale, turn to the right, and grasp the sides of the chair back with your hands. If your feet are not comfortably on the floor, place a folded blanket or phone book under them.
3. As you inhale, bring your back up tall as if you were trying to touch the ceiling with the top of your spine.
4. As you exhale twist your torso and head farther to the right.
5. Return to the starting position. Repeat the twist, gradually twisting farther with each exhalation for 3 breaths, but do not go beyond your comfort zone. On the last repetition, hold the twist for 4 to 6 breaths; then return to the starting position.
6. Repeat the same sequence on the opposite side.

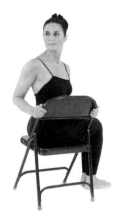

Standing Forward Bend with Chair

This movement stretches the backside of your body, including upper and lower back, neck, and hamstrings.

1. Stand with your feet hip-width apart, arm's distance from the seat of a chair. Keep the spine tall but relaxed. Let your arms hang at your sides, palms turned inward toward your legs. Look straight ahead.
2. As you inhale, raise your arms to the front, up and overhead.
3. As you exhale, slowly bend forward from the hips, bringing your arms, hands, torso, and head forward and down until the palms touch the front edge of the chair. Slightly bend your knees.
4. As you inhale, return to the upright position, keeping your arms raised.
5. Repeat 3 times. Then stay in Step 3 in the forward bend position for 6 to 8 breaths. Slowly return to the upright position.

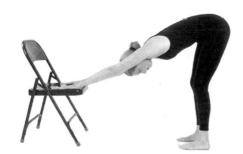

Balancing Cat

This posture helps improve your overall balance and stability.

1. Start on your hands and knees with the heels of your hands directly below your shoulders, your knees at hip width.
2. As you exhale, slowly slide your right hand forward and your left leg backward as far as they will go on the ground. Pause briefly.
3. As you inhale, raise your right hand and left leg up as high as you feel comfortable, or until they are both parallel to the floor. As you exhale, bring them both down to the floor, keeping them in the extended position.
4. Repeat the lifting motion 3 times; then hold in the lifted position for 4 to 6 breaths.
5. Repeat the sequence with your left arm and right leg.

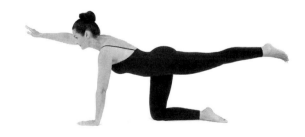

Lying Leg and Arm Raise with Bent Legs

This exercise gently stretches the hamstrings and the upper and lower back, while toning the abdomen.

1. Lie on your back with your arms at your sides. Bend both knees and bring them toward your chest.
2. As you inhale, slowly bring your arms straight up and back, while raising your legs. Keep going until your arms are touching the ground behind you, and your legs are straight up, with the knees slightly bent.
3. As you exhale, return to the starting position.
4. Repeat 6 to 8 times.

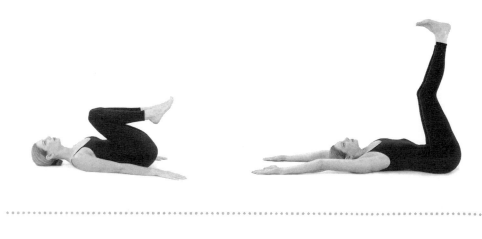

Bridge

This posture promotes circulation to the neck and shoulders, and strengthens the back, shoulders, hips, and thighs.

1. Lie on your back, bend your knees, and place your feet on the floor at hip width.
2. Relax your arms at your sides, palms down.
3. As you inhale, use your abdominal muscles to raise your hips halfway up. Pause. Then lift your hips as high as you feel comfortable. Do not go past halfway if it causes you any back pain.
4. As you exhale, bring your hips back to the floor.
5. Repeat 6 to 8 times, remembering to pause halfway up.

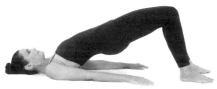

Bent-Leg Corpse

This is the classic posture for relaxation, with bent legs to support your back.

1. Lie on your back with your arms at your sides, palms up. Place pillows or rolled blankets under your knees for comfort.
2. Bend your knees with your feet flat on the floor, at hip width. If your head tilts back or your throat is tense, use a pillow or folded blanket under your head. Stay in this position for 6 to 8 breaths.
3. Relax with your eyes closed.

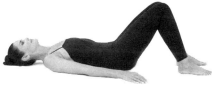

Alternate Nostril Breathing

This technique helps to create balance and harmony in your system. It is described in detail on page 45. Do 10 to 12 cycles, sitting comfortably in a chair or on the floor.

Meditation

1. Remain seated comfortably in a chair or on the floor.
2. Use Focused (page 57), Open-Ended (page 58), or Mantra (page 59) Meditation for at least 5 minutes.

Breathing Break

Once per day, take a break to practice Alternate Nostril Breathing (page 45) for five to ten minutes.

Affirmation

You may want to compose your own affirmation that applies directly to your situation. Repeat your affirmation upon rising and on retiring at night; before all meals; and whenever you start to have cravings, negative thoughts, or fears throughout the day. If you like, you can use the following affirmation: "Every day, in every way, I grow stronger, with my body, breath, and mind."

Appendix A

RESOURCE GUIDE

The Bibliography (page 281) lists highly recommended books about Yoga and healing. The following is a list of resources to help you further explore Yoga, holistic health, and specific ailments. Please feel free to contact us at our Web site, www.samata.com.

GENERAL INFORMATION ON YOGA AND HOLISTIC HEALING

Yoga Research and Education Center/International Association
   of Yoga Therapists
2400-A County Center Dr.
Santa Rosa, CA 95403
707-566-9000
Web sites: www.yrec.org, www.iayt.org

Yoga Journal: www.yogajournal.com

Roots and Wings: www.yoga.com

Holistic-online: www.holisticonline.com

WebMD: www.webmd.com

Helios Health: www.helioshealth.com

All Experts: www.allexperts.com

The Merck Manual Home Edition: www.merckhomeedition.com

U.S. Centers for Disease Control and Prevention: www.cdc.gov

American Academy of Family Physicians: familydoctor.org

VIDEOS AND MUSIC

Larry Payne's User Friendly Yoga (VHS tapes) (www.samata.com)

You can find music for Yoga in the New Age section of your local music or video store. While we have dozens of favorites, here are some CDs we recommend.

Spectrum Suite or *Music for Yoga* by Steven Halpern, Inner Peace Music (widely available)

Buddha or *Santosh* by P. C. Davidoff and Friends, Garland of Letters
 (www.garlandofletters.com)

Adagio Music for Yoga by Peter Davison, Living Arts (widely available)

Mariner or *Rainforest Magic* by Tony O'Connor (www.tonyoconnor.com.au)

RESOURCES BY CHAPTER

Chapter 1: How Yoga Heals

BOOKS

How to Know God, The Yoga Aphorisms of Patanjali. Translated by Swami Prabhavananda
 and Christopher Isherwood. The Vedanta Society of Southern California, 1981.

Dorothy Gault-McNemee. *God's Diet: A Short and Simple Way to Eat Naturally, Lose
 Weight, and Live a Healthier Life.* Three Rivers Press, 2000.

Andrew Weil. *Spontaneous Healing: How to Discover and Embrace Your Body's Natural Ability to Maintain and Heal Itself.* Ballantine Books, 2000.

Sherry Brourman, R.P.T. *Walk Yourself Well.* Hyperion, 1999.

Chapter 3: Getting Started with Yoga Therapy

Where to Buy Yoga Props

Hugger Mugger Yoga Props
and Products
31 West Gregson Ave.
Salt Lake City, UT 84115
800-473-4888

Body Slant
Gravity Inversion Tools
P.O. Box 1667
Newport Beach, CA 92663
800-443-3917

More Yoga
7603 Granada Dr.
Bethesda, MD 20817
888-MRE-YOGA (888-667-7642)
E-mail: info@moreyoga.com

Invertebod
International Sports Medicine Institute
3283 Motor Ave.
West Los Angeles, CA 90034
(800)-Bad-Back (800 223-2225)

Chapter 4: The Wind in Your Sails

Books

Donna Farhi. *The Breathing Book: Good Health and Vitality through Essential Breath Work.* Henry Holt, 1996.

B. K. S. Iyengar. *Light on Pranayama: The Yogic Art of Breathing.* Crossroad/Herder & Herder, 1995.

Chapter 5: Relaxation and Meditation

Books

Larry Rosenberg with David Guy. *Breath by Breath: The Liberating Practice of Insight Meditation.* Shambhala Publications, Inc., 1999.

Richard C. Miller. *Mudra: Gateways to Self-Understanding.* Available from www.nondual.com.

Richard C. Miller. *The Principles and Practice of Yoga Nidra*. Available from www.nondual.com.

Shinzen Young. *Beginner's Mind*. Available from www.shinzen.org.

Instruction in meditation from the Worldwide Online Meditation Center, www.meditationcenter.com

Chapter 7: The Musculoskeletal System

Books

Art Brownstein. *Healing Back Pain Naturally*. Harbor Press, 1999.

John Sarno. *Mind Over Back Pain*. Berkley Books, 1999.

Robert Forster, P.T., and Lynda Huey, M.A. *The Water Power Workout*. Random House, 1993.

Ron Lawrence, M.D., Ph.D., and Martin Zucker. *Preventing Arthritis*. Putnam, 2001.

Web Sites

Spine Health: www.spine-health.com

Arthritis Foundation: www.arthritis.org

Chapter 8: The Respiratory System

Books

Ellen W. Cutler. *Winning the War against Immune Disorders and Allergies: A Drug Free Cure for Allergies*. Delmar, 1998.

Web Sites

American Academy of Allergy, Asthma, and Immunology: www.aaaai.org

Asthma and Allergy Foundation of America: www.aafa.org

Chapter 9: The Circulatory System

Books

Dean Ornish. *Dr. Dean Ornish's Program for Reversing Heart Disease*. Ivy Books, 1996.

Peter O. Kwiterovich. *Johns Hopkins Complete Guide to Preventing and Reversing Heart Disease.* Prima Publishing, 1998.

Web Sites

American Heart Association: www.americanheart.org
National Stroke Association: www.stroke.org

Chapter 10: The Digestive System

Books

Sherry A. Rogers. *No More Heartburn: Stop the Pain in 30 Days—Naturally!* Kensington, 2000.
D. Lindsey Berkson. *Healthy Digestion the Natural Way.* John Wiley, 2000.

Web Sites

The Mind-Body Digestive Center: www.mindbodydigestive.com
National Institute of Diabetes and Digestive and Kidney Diseases: www.niddk.nih.gov.

Chapter 11: The Nervous System

Books

Seymour Diamond. *Coping with Your Headaches.* International Universities Press, 1988.
Barbara Moe. *Everything You Need to Know about Migraines and Other Headaches.* Rosen Publishing Group, 2000.

Web Sites

National Headache Foundation: www.headaches.org
American Council for Headache Education: www.achenet.org

Chapter 12: For Women Only

Books

Christiane Northrup. *The Wisdom of Menopause.* Bantam Doubleday Dell, 2001.
Gail Sheehy. *The Silent Passage: Menopause.* Pocket Books, 1998.

Carol Landau, Michele G. Cyr, Anne W. Moulton. *The Complete Book of Menopause: Every Woman's Guide to Health*. Perigee, 1995.

Web Sites

National Women's Health Information Center: www.4woman.gov
Yoga and Menopause: www.hotflashyoga.com
American College of Obsetricians and Gynecologists: www.acog.org

Chapter 13: Mental Health

Books

Andrew Solomon. *The Noonday Demon: An Atlas of Depression*. Scribner, 2001.
Edmund J. Bourne. *Beyond Anxiety and Phobia: A Step-By-Step Guide to Lifetime Recovery*. New Harbinger Publications, 2001.

Web Sites

National Mental Health Association: www.nmha.org
American Psychological Association: http://helping.apa.org

Chapter 14: Endocrine System

American Diabetes Association: 800-Diabetes (800-342-2383)
  Web site: www.diabetes.org

Books

Hope S. Warshaw. *Diabetes Meal Planning Made Easy*. McGraw-Hill, 1996.
Barbara C. Hansen, Shauna S. Roberts. *The Commonsense Guide to Weight Loss (For People with Diabetes)*. McGraw-Hill, 1998.
Dean Ornish. *Everyday Cooking with Dr. Dean Ornish: 150 Easy, Low-Fat, High-Flavor Recipes*. HarperCollins, 1997.
Judy Wardell. *Thin Within: How to Eat and Live Like a Thin Person*. Crown, 1997.

Appendix B

FINDING A YOGA THERAPIST

IN YOUR AREA

The Yoga information in this book is inspired by the teachings of T. K. V. Desikachar of Chennai (formerly Madras), India. He and his father, the late Professor T. Krishnamacharya, developed the style of Yoga known as Viniyoga. This style emphasizes practicing postures, breathing, and meditation according to your individual needs and capacity, as opposed to achieving ideal external form. For information about a Viniyoga instructor in your area contact one of the following centers for a referral.

American Viniyoga Institute
Gary and Mirka Kraftsow
P.O. Box 88
Makawao, HI 96768
808-572-1414
E-mail: info@viniyoga.com
Web site: www.viniyoga.com

Antaranga Yoga Center
Sonia Nelson
PMB 131
1704 Llano St., Suite B
Santa Fe, NM 87505
505-982-3308
Web site: vedicchantcenter.org

Pierce Yoga Program
Margaret Pierce
1164 North Highland Ave., NE
Atlanta, GA 30306
404-875-7110
E-mail: pierceyoga@mindspring.com
Web site: www.pierceyoga.com

Samata Yoga Center
Larry Payne, Ph.D.
4150 Tivoli Ave.
Los Angeles, CA 90066
800-359-0171
E-mail: samata@aol.com
Web site: www.samata.com

INTERNATIONAL

Viniyoga Britain
Paul Harvey
105 Gales Drive, Three Bridges, Crawley
West Sussex RH10 1QD, U.K.
Phone: 01 293 53664
Email: info@viniyoga.co.uk
Web site: www.viniyoga.co.uk

KYM
Krishnamacharya Yoga Mandiram
New No.31 (Old #13) Fourth Cross Street
R K Nagar, Chennai–600 028, India.
Phone: 91.44.4937998
E-mail: admin@kym.org
Web site: www.kym.org

Formation Viniyoga
Bernard Bouanchaud
17 rue Elisee Reclus
91120 Palaiseau, France
Phone: 01 60 10 78 81
E-mail:aagamaat@wanadoo.fr

Appendix C

FIGURING YOUR BODY MASS INDEX (BMI)

TO CALCULATE YOUR BMI

1. Multiply your weight (in pounds) by 704.5 (Write it down.)
2. Multiply your height in inches by itself. (Write it down.)
3. Divide the first result by the second.

4. The resulting number is your BMI.

TO INTERPRET THE RESULTS

18.5 or below: underweight

18.5 to 24.9: healthy weight

25 to 29.9: overweight

30 or above: obese

Example

For a person who is 5 feet, 4 inches (64 inches) and weighs 130 pounds:

$130 \times 704.5 = 91,585$

$64 \times 64 = 4,096$

$91,585 \div 4,096 = 22.36$ (BMI)

A BMI of 22.36 means this person is of a healthy weight.

Notes

Chapter 7

1. U.S. Centers for Disease Control and Prevention. "Arthritis: The Nation's Leading Cause of Disability." Online: www.cdc.gov/nccdphp/arthritis/index.htm.

2. Marian S. Garfinkel and H. R. Schumacher Jr. "Yoga." *Rheumatic Diseases Clinics of North America* 26, no. 1 (2000): 125–32.

3. U.S. Centers for Disease Control and Prevention. "Facts About Arthritis." Online: www.cdc.gov/od/oc/media/fact/arthriti.htm.

4. David Yocum, Les Castro, and Michelle Cornett. "Exercise, Education, and Behavioral Modification as Alternative Therapy for Pain and Stress in Rheumatic Disease." *Rheumatic Diseases Clinics of North America* 26, no. 1 (2000): 145–59.

5. T. V. Ananthanarayanan and T. M. Srinivasan. "Asana Based Exercises for the Management of Low Back Pain." *The Yoga Review* 3, no. 1 (1983): 45–58. Reprinted in *Journal of the International Association of Yoga Therapists* (1994): 6–15.

Chapter 8

1. American Academy of Allergy, Asthma and Immunology. "Patient/Public Education: Fast Facts: Myth vs. Reality." Online: www.aaaai.com/patients/resources/fastfacts/mythvsreality.stm.

2. Jackie Joyner-Kersee. "Asthma and the Athlete's Challenge." *New York Times,* August 13, 2001. Sec. A, p. 17, Col. 2.

3. Dee Ann Birkel and Lee Edgren. "Hatha Yoga: Improved Vital Capacity of College Students." *Alternative Therapies in Health and Medicine* 6, no. 6 (2000): 55–63.

4. The following studies showed that asthmatic patients improved after doing Yoga:
• P. K. Vedanthan et al. "Clinical Study of Yoga Techniques in University Students with Asthma: A Controlled Study." Northern Colorado Allergy Asthma Clinic, Fort Collins. *Allergy and Asthma Proceedings: The Official Journal of Regional and State Allergy Societies* 19, no. 1 (1998): 3–9. • A. A. Khanam et al. "Study of Pulmonary and Autonomic Functions of Asthma Patients after Yoga Training." All India Institute of Medical Science, New Delhi. *Indian Journal of Physiology and Pharmacology* 40, no. 4 (1976): 318–324. • S. C. Jain et al. "Effect of Yoga Training on Exercise Tolerance in Adolescents with Childhood Asthma." Central Research Institute for Yoga, New Delhi. *Journal of Asthma,* 28, no. 6 (1991): 437–442. • V. Singh et al. "Effect of Yoga Breathing Exercises (Pranayama) on Airway Reactivity in Subjects with Asthma." Respiratory Medicine Unit, City Hospital, Nottingham, UK. *Lancet* 335, no. 8702 (1990): 1381–1383.

5. H. R. Nagendra et al. "An Integrated Approach of Yoga Therapy for Bronchial Asthma: A 3–54-Month Prospective Study." *Journal of Asthma* 23, no. 3 (1986): 123–137.

6. R. Nagarathna and H. R. Nagendra. "Yoga for Bronchial Asthma: A Controlled Study." *British Medical Journal (Clinical Research Edition)* 291, no. 6502 (1985): 1077–1079.

7. Barbara O. Rennard, et al. "Chicken Soup Inhibits Neutrophil Chemotaxis *In Vitro.*" *Chest* 118 (2000): 1150–1157.

Chapter 9

1. Well-Connected Board of Editors, Harvey Simon, Editor-in-Chief. "How Serious Is High Blood Pressure?" Online: WebMD, March 1999, my.webmd.com/content/article/1680.50586.

2. According to National Stroke Association. Online: www.stroke.org/stroke_risk.cfm.

3. National Institutes of Health. *The Sixth Report of the Joint National Committee on Prevention, Detection and Evaluation and Treatment of High Blood Pressure* [NIH Publication No. 98-4080]. National Heart, Lung, and Blood Institute, National High Blood Pressure Education Program, November 1997.

4. American Heart Association. "Atherosclerosis: What Is Atherosclerosis?" Online: 216.185.112.5/presenter.jhtml?identifier=4440.

5. American Heart Association. "About Sudden Death and Cardiac Arrest." Online: www.americanheart.org/presenter.jhtml?identifier=604

6. Donna L. Hoyert et al. "Deaths: Final Data for 1999." U.S. Centers for Disease Control and Prevention. *National Vital Statistics Reports* 49, no. 8 (2001): 1–114.

7. K. K. Datey et al. "Shavasan: A Yogic Exercise in the Management of Hypertension." *Angiology* 20, no. 6 (1969): 325–333.

8. S. Sundar et al. "Role of Yoga in Management of Essential Hypertension." *Acta Cardiologica* 39, no. 3 (1984): 203–208.

9. R. Murugesan, N. Govindarajulu, and T. K. Bera. "Effect of Selected Yogic Practices on the Management of Hypertension." *Indian Journal of Physiology and Pharmacology* 44, no. 2 (2000): 207–210.

10. M. P. Anand. "Non-Pharmacological Management of Essential Hypertension." *Journal of the Indian Medical Association* 97, no. 6 (1999): 220–225.

11. A. G. Mohan, Ron Accomazzo, Arthur Petyan, and Marsha Accomazzo. Unpublished study commissioned by the **International Association of Yoga Therapists** (1990).

12. Dean Ornish, et al. "Intensive Lifestyle Changes for Reversal of Coronary Heart Disease." *Journal of the American Medical Association* 280, no. 23 (1998): 2001–2007.

13. S. C. Manchanda et al. "Retardation of Coronary Atherosclerosis with Yoga Lifestyle Intervention." *The Journal of the Association of Physicians of India* 48, no. 7 (2000): 687–694.

14. A. S. Mahajan, K. S. Reddy, and U. Sachdeva. "Lipid Profile of Coronary Risk Subjects Following Yogic Lifestyle Intervention." *Indian Heart Journal* 51, no. 1 (1999): 37–40.

Chapter 10

General information for this chapter was provided by the National Digestive Diseases Information Clearinghouse, a service of the National Institute of Diabetes and Digestive and

Kidney Diseases (NIDDK). NIDDK is part of the National Institutes of Health under the U.S. Public Health Service.

1. This comes from the ancient Yoga text *The Upanishads,* a series of mystical discourses that are part of the *Vedas,* considered the most sacred scripture of Hinduism.
2. Charles Gerson and Mary Joan Gerson. "IBS Information: The Mind and the Body." Online: *The Mind Body Digestive Center,* New York, www.mindbodydigestive.com/.
3. National Digestive Diseases Information Clearinghouse. *Ulcerative Colitis* [NIH Publication No. 95-1597]. NIDDK, April 1992.
4. Robin Monro, R. Nagarathna, and H. R. Nagendra. *Yoga for Common Ailments.* New York: Simon & Schuster, 1990.
5. Well-Connected Board of Editors, Harvey Simon, Editor-in-Chief. "Who Gets Gastroesophageal Reflux Disease?" Online: WebMD, March 1999, my.webmd.com/condition_center_content/hbn/article/1680.51292.
6. Gary Kraftsow. *Yoga for Wellness.* New York: Penguin Putnam, 1999.

Chapter 11

1. *Migraine: The Complete Guide.* Mt. Royal, NJ: American Council for Headache Education, 1994.
2. U.S. Food and Drug Administration. "Heading Off Migraine Pain." Online: May–June 1998, www.fda.gov/fdac/features/1998/398_pain.html.
3. Dean Ornish. "Ask Dr. Ornish: Q&A." Online: WebMD, my.webmd.com/content/article/3079.632.
4. Robin Monroe. *Yoga for Common Ailments.* New York: Simon & Schuster, 1990.

Chapter 12

General information for this chapter was provided by the U.S. Department of Health and Human Services, the U.S. Food and Drug Administration (www.fda.gov), and MedicineNet.com (an online health-care media publishing company).

1. Well-Connected Board of Editors, Harvey Simon, Editor-in-Chief. "How Serious Is Premenstrual Syndrome?" Online: WebMD, September 2000, my.webmd.com/content/article/1680.53171.

2. Louise Wiggins. "Menopause and Yoga." *International Light: The Official Journal of the International Yoga Teachers Association* (July–September 1999).

3. The Pennsylvania State University's Women's Health. "Disease & Health Information: Menopause." The Milton S. Hershey Medical Center, The Penn State University. Online: www.hmc.psu.edu/healthinfo/m/menopause.htm.

Chapter 13

1. American Psychiatric Association. "Generalized Anxiety Disorder." In *Diagnostic and Statistical Manual of Mental Disorders (DSM-IV)*. Washington, D.C.: American Psychiatric Press, 1994, pp. 432–36.

2. American Psychiatric Association. "Panic Disorder." In *Diagnostic and Statistical Manual of Mental Disorders (DSM-IV)*. Washington, D.C.: American Psychiatric Press, 1994, pp. 397–403.

3. American Psychiatric Association. "Post Traumatic Stress Disorder (PTSD)." In *Diagnostic and Statistical Manual of Mental Disorders (DSM IV)*. Washington, D.C.: American Psychiatric Press, 1994, pp. 424–29.

4. Carol Ann Turkington and Eliot F. Kaplan. "What is Depression?" Online: WebMD, http//my.webmd.com/content/article/1680.50544. From *Making the Prozac Decision: A Guide to Antidepressants.* 3rd ed. New York: McGraw Hill, 1997.

5. American Psychiatric Association. "Depression." In *Diagnostic and Statistical Manual of Mental Disorders (DSM-IV)*, Washington, D.C.: American Psychiatric Press, 1994, pp. 339–45.

6. Turkington and Kaplan, *op.cit.*

7. Alice Christensen. *The American Yoga Association Wellness Book*. Kensington Books, 1997.

8. John H. Greist, et al. "Running as Treatment for Depression." *Comprehensive Psychiatry* 20, no. 1 (1979): 41–54.

9. U.S. Ray et al. "Effect of Yogic Exercises on Physical and Mental Health of Young Fellowship Course Trainees." *Indian Journal of Physiology and Pharmacology* 45, no. 1 (2001): 37–53.

10. A. Malathi and A. Damodaran. "Stress Due to Exams in Medical Students—Role of Yoga." *Indian Journal of Physiology and Pharmacology* 43, no. 2 (1999): 218–224.

11. J. J. Miller, K. Fletcher, and J. Kabat-Zinn. "Three-year Follow Up and Clinical Implications of a Mindfulness Meditation–Based Stress Reduction Intervention in the Treatment of Anxiety Disorders." *General Hospital Psychiatry* 17, no. 3 (1995): 192–200.

Chapter 14

1. U.S. Centers for Disease Control and Prevention. "Press Release: Twin Epidemics of Diabetes and Obesity Continue to Threaten the Health of Americans, CDC Says." Online: September 11, 2001, www.cdc.gov/nccdphp/dnpa/press/twinepid.htm.
2. American Diabetes Association. Online: www.diabetes.org.
3. D. Gallagher et al. "Healthy Percentage Body Fat Ranges: An Approach for Developing Guidelines Based on Body Mass Index." *American Journal of Clinical Nutrition* 72, no. 3 (2000): 694–701.
4. R. S. Surwit et al. "Stress Management Improves Long-term Glycemic Control in Type 2 Diabetes." *Diabetes Care* 25, no. 1 (2002): 30–34.

Bibliography

All of the books in this list have been immensely helpful to us in writing this book, and we thank their authors for their tremendous contributions to our understanding of Yoga's healing properties.

American Psychiatric Association. *Diagnostic and Statistical Manual of Mental Disorders (DSM-IV)*. Washington, D.C.: American Psychiatric Press, 1994.

Balch, Phyllis A., and James F. Balch. *Prescription for Nutritional Healing.* 3rd ed. New York: Avery, 2000.

Carrico, Mara, and the editors of *Yoga Journal. Yoga Journal's Yoga Basics.* New York: Henry Holt, 1997.

Christensen, Alice. *The American Yoga Association Wellness Book.* New York: Kensington Books, 1996.

Desikachar, T. K. V. *The Heart of Yoga: Developing a Personal Practice.* Rochester, VT: Inner Traditions, 1995.

Desikachar, T. K. V. with Kausthub Desikachar and Frans Moors. *The Viniyoga of Yoga.* *Chenna,* Quandra Press, 2001.

Desikachar, T. K. V. and Arjun Rajagopalan. *The Yoga of Healing.* Chennai, India: Eastwest Books, 1999.

Devi, Nischala Joy. *The Healing Path of Yoga.* New York: Three Rivers, 2000.

Feuerstein, Georg. *Encyclopedic Dictionary of Yoga.* New York: Paragon, 1990.

————. *The Shambhala Encyclopedia of Yoga.* Boston: Shambhala, 1997.

Feuerstein, Georg, and Larry Payne. *Yoga for Dummies.* Foster City, CA: IDG Books, 1999.

Huey, Lynda, and Robert Forster. *The Complete Waterpower Workout Book.* New York: Random House, 1993.

Iyengar, B. K. S. *Yoga: The Path to Holistic Health.* London: Dorling Kindersley, 2001.

Karmananda Saraswati, Swami. *Yogic Management of Common Diseases.* Bihar, India: Bihar School of Yoga, 1979.

Klapper, Robert, and Lynda Huey. *Heal Your Hips.* New York: John Wiley, 1999.

Kraftsow, Gary. *Yoga for Wellness.* New York: Penguin Putnam, 1999.

Krishnamacharya, Yogacarya T. *Sri Nathamuni's Yogarahasya.* Translated by T. K. V. Desikachar. Chennai, India: Krishnamacharya Yoga Mandiram, 1998.

Krucoff, Carol, and Mitchell Krucoff. *Healing Moves.* New York: Harmony Books, 2000.

Kuvalayananda, Swami. *Pranayama.* India: Kaivalyadhama, Lonavla, 1977.

Kuvalayananda, Swami, and S. L. Vinekar. *Yogic Therapy.* New Delhi, India: Indian Ministry of Health and Family Welfare, 1994.

Lawrence, Ronald M., and Martin Zucker. *Preventing Arthritis: A Holistic Approach to Life without Pain.* New York: Putnam, 2001.

Mohan, A. G. *Yoga for Body, Breath and Mind: A Guide to Personal Reintegration.* Portland, OR: Rudra Press, 1993.

Monro, Robin, with R. Nagarathna and H. R. Nagendra. *Yoga for Common Ailments.* New York: Simon & Schuster, 1990.

Oz, Mehmet. *Healing from the Heart*. New York: Plume, 1999.

Pierce, Margaret D., and Martin G. Pierce. *Yoga for Your Life*. Portland, OR: Rudra Press, 1996.

Polk, Irwin J. *All about Asthma: Stop Suffering and Start Living*. New York: Insight Books, 1997.

Raman, Krishna. *A Matter of Health: Integration of Yoga and Western Medicine for Prevention and Cure*. Chennai, India: Eastwest Books, 1998.

Sarno, John. *Healing Back Pain: The Mind-Body Connection*. New York: Warner Books, 1991.

Satchidananda, Swami. *Integral Yoga Hatha*. New York: Holt, Rinehart & Winston, 1970.

Satyananda Saraswati, Swami. *Asana Pranayama Mudra Bandha*. Bihar, India: Bihar School of Yoga, 1973.

Shankardevananda Saraswati, Swami. *The Effects of Yoga on Hypertension*. Bihar, India: Bihar School of Yoga, 1984.

———. *The Practices of Yoga for the Digestive System*. Bihar, India: Bihar School of Yoga, 1979.

Shankardevananda Saraswati, Swami. *Yogic Management of Asthma and Diabetes*. Bihar, India: Bihar School of Yoga, 1979.

Sinel, Michael, and William W. Deardorff. *Back Pain Remedies for Dummies*. Foster City, CA: IDG Books, 1999.

Stiles, Mukunda. *Structural Yoga Therapy: Adapting to the Individual*. York Beach, ME: Weiser, 2000.

Swezey, Robert L., and Annette M. Swezey. *Good News for Bad Backs*. Santa Monica, CA: Cequal, 1993.

Van Lysebeth, Andre. *Pranayama: The Yoga of Breathing*. London: Unwin, 1979.

Vishnudevananda, Swami. *The Complete Illustrated Book of Yoga*. New York: Pocket Books, 1960.

Weller, Stella. *Yoga Therapy*. London: HarperCollins, 1995.

Quick Reference to Postures, Breathing,

Relaxation, and Meditation

Index

Note: Postures, breathing exercises, relaxation and meditation techniques are also listed separately in the Quick Reference on page 285.

bursae, 99
bursitis, 108

cancer, 102
capsaicin, 113
carpal tunnel syndrome, 108
cartilage, 105, 110
channel of comfort, 50
Chest-to-Belly Breathing, 42, 78, 231,
    238, 246
chicken soup, 160
Child's Posture, 73
cholesterol, 9, 173–75
chondroitin sulfate, 113
circulation, 7, 19, 21,
    Yoga view of, 30, 104
circulatory system, 173–74
Cobra, 122, 243
    (Kite Variation), 72
cognitive-behavioral therapy, 233–34,
    236
cold season, 156
colon, 191. See also bowels
commitment, 24, 55
common cold, 153
    definition of, 156
    frequency of, 156
    testimonial, 159
    Yoga Prescription for, 160
    Yoga Routine for, 171
    Yoga view of, 157
compensation, 30
competition, 29
concentration, 20
Cooling Breath, 47, 230
Core Routine I, 62
Core Routine II, 78
Corpse, 70, 85, 171
    Bent-Legs, 114, 137, 262
    Bent-Leg with Long Exhale, 127, 201
    (Supported) with Belly Breathing, 188,
        201, 217
    with Blankets, 230, 246
    with Yoga Nidra, 247

coronary artery disease (CAD), 9, 175–76
    Yoga Prescription for, 179
    Yoga Routine for, 188
    See also heart disease
Crow's Beak, 47, 230
culture, 23–24

degenerative joint disease, 107
    See also osteoarthritis
depression, 232, 234
    major, 234–35
    Yoga Prescription for, 237
    Yoga Routine for, 238
Desikachar, Kaustab, 18
Desikachar, T.K.V., xiii, 42, 109
deviated septum, 38
diabetes, 249–50, 251–52
    type 1, 250
    type 2, 250, 252
    Yoga Prescription for, 254
    Yoga Routine for, 256
diaphragm, 35–36
diet
    calcium and, 112
    diabetes and, 251
    digestive problems and, 192, 194
    headaches and, 207
    heart disease and, 180
    obesity and, 252
    respiratory ailments and, 152, 153, 158
    Yoga approach to, 9–11
digestion, 10
digestive system, 191
discipline
    developing, 253
    in Yoga practice, 24
    self-, 6, 7
    Yoga definition and, 5
disks, intervertebral, 99, 100, 103
    illus. 103
duodenum, 191
dynamic and static, 27, 29
dysmenorrhea, 220. See also menstrual
    cramps

About the Authors

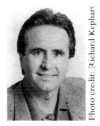

Photo credit: Richard Kephart

LARRY PAYNE, PH.D., is an internationally prominent Yoga teacher and workshop leader specializing in back problems. He is the coauthor of *Yoga for Dummies* and author of *The Business of Teaching Yoga*. During his previous career as an advertising sales executive, Yoga helped Dr. Payne overcome his own back problems.

Based in Los Angeles, Dr. Payne is director of the Samata Yoga Center, cofounder of the Yoga program at the University of California at Los Angeles School of Medicine, and director of the International Association of Yoga Therapists. He is also founder of the corporate Yoga program at the J. Paul Getty Museum and has created similar programs for Rancho La Puerta Fitness Spa, The Ritz Carlton and Loews Hotels, and numerous other corporations. Dr. Payne has received Outstanding Achievement Awards for Yoga in Europe, South America, and the United States and has been featured on CNN, national TV shows, and syndicated radio programs. He has also been featured in the *New York Times* and the *Los Angeles Times* as well as numerous international publications.

Dr. Payne conducts a private Yoga therapy practice in Marina del Rey and Malibu, California. In addition to speaking engagements and workshops, he is featured in the "User Friendly Yoga" video series. His Web site is www.Samata.com.

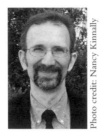

RICHARD P. USATINE, M.D., is a family physician, teacher, and author. He is Associate Dean for Medical Education at the new Florida State University (FSU) College of Medicine. Dr. Usatine received his medical degree from Columbia University College of Physicians and Surgeons and completed his family medicine residency at University of California at Los Angeles (UCLA) Medical Center. He was the first full-time medical director of the Venice Family Clinic, one of the largest free clinics in the U.S. Dr. Usatine was the producer and host of the Los Angeles cable TV show *To Your Health*.

In 1989, Dr. Usatine became Associate Director of the UCLA Family Medicine Residency Training Program and subsequently served as Assistant Dean of Student Affairs at the UCLA School of Medicine. He was a co-founder of the Doctoring Curriculum and is dedicated to teaching doctors to communicate effectively with their patients. His work with homeless families has been featured on the Discovery Health Channel.

In 2000, Dr. Usatine was honored to receive the Humanism in Medical Education award from the Association of American Medical Colleges, which annually honors one medical school faculty physician for embodying the finest qualities in a healer. Dr. Usatine was recruited from UCLA to help start the first new medical school in the country in over twenty years. He is leading the development of a new state-of-the-art twenty-first-century medical curriculum at Florida State University. He is committed to training compassionate caring physicians and bringing quality health care to everyone including the underserved communities of the world.